Second hand tobacco smoke kills 600 000 people each year

There is no safe level of exposure to second-hand tobacco smoke.

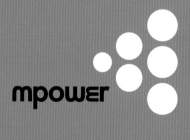

mpower

Monitor	Monitor tobacco use and prevention policies
Protect	Protect people from tobacco smoke
Offer	Offer help to quit tobacco use
Warn	Warn about the dangers of tobacco
Enforce	Enforce bans on tobacco advertising, promotion and sponsorship
Raise	Raise taxes on tobacco

Globally, about one third of adults are regularly exposed to second-hand tobacco smoke.

WHO Report on the Global Tobacco Epidemic, 2009: Implementing smoke-free environments is the second in a series of WHO reports that tracks the status of the tobacco epidemic and the impact of interventions implemented to stop it.

WHO Library Cataloguing-in-Publication Data

WHO report on the global tobacco epidemic, 2009:
implementing smoke-free environments.

    1.Smoking - prevention and control. 2.Tobacco smoke
    pollution - prevention and control. 3.Tobacco smoke
    pollution - legislation and jurisprudence. 4.Health policy.
    I.World Health Organization.

ISBN 978 92 4 156391 8   (NLM classification: WM 290)

Printed in France

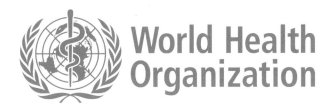
World Health Organization

WHO REPORT ON THE GLOBAL TOBACCO EPIDEMIC, 2009

Implementing smoke-free environments

Made possible by funding from Bloomberg Philanthropies

Contents

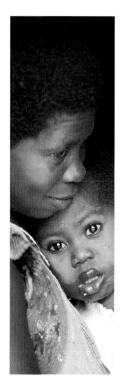
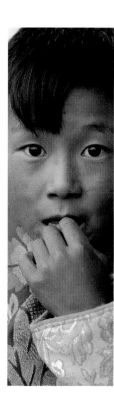
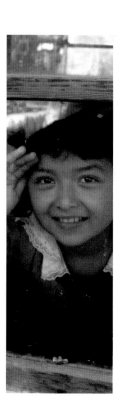
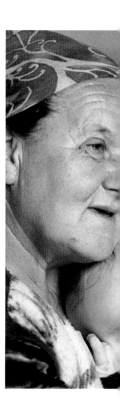

Appendices IV through X are available in electronic format on the CD accompanying this book and online at www.who.int/tobacco/mpower/en.

ABBREVIATIONS

AFR	**WHO Regional Office for Africa**
AMR	**WHO Regional Office for the Americas**
CDC	**Centers for Disease Control and Prevention**
COP	**Conference of the Parties**
EMR	**WHO Regional Office for the Eastern Mediterranean**
EUR	**WHO Regional Office for Europe**
NRT	**Nicotine Replacement Therapy**
SEAR	**WHO Regional Office for South-East Asia**
STEPS	**WHO's STEPwise approach to Surveillance**
US$	**United States dollar**
WHO	**World Health Organization**
WHO FCTC	**WHO Framework Convention on Tobacco Control**
WPR	**WHO Regional Office for the Western Pacific**

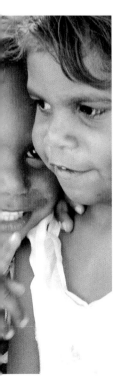
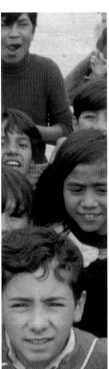
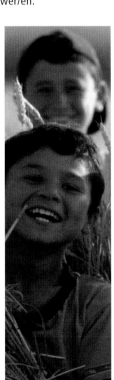
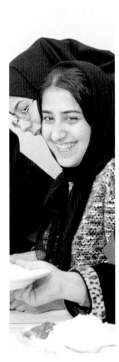

Despite progress, only 9% of countries mandate smoke-free bars and restaurants, and 65 countries report no implementation of any smoke-free policies on a national level.

Governments around the world, in partnership with civil society, must continue to act decisively against the tobacco epidemic – the leading global cause of preventable death.

Dr Ala Alwan, Assistant Director-General, World Health Organization

PROGRESS IS BEING MADE – NEARLY 400 MILLION PEOPLE NEWLY COVERED BY TOBACCO CONTROL MEASURES IN 2008

Since the entry into force of the WHO Framework Convention on Tobacco Control (WHO FCTC), we have made considerable progress against the global tobacco epidemic. Through results presented in this *WHO Report on the Global Tobacco Epidemic, 2009* – the second country-level examination of the global tobacco epidemic – we know which countries have implemented effective tobacco control measures to reduce demand for tobacco, which countries need to do more to protect their people against the harms of tobacco use, and which countries can be held up as models for action.

Tobacco use continues to kill more than 5 million people worldwide each year, and this number is expected to grow. The burden of tobacco use is greatest in low- and middle-income countries, and will increase more rapidly in these countries in coming decades. We must continue to expand and intensify our efforts to reduce tobacco use.

Tobacco control is relatively inexpensive to implement, and the return is enormous. Tobacco use kills or disables many people in their most productive years, which denies families their primary wage-earners, consumes family budgets, raises the cost of health care and hinders economic development. While there are some costs associated with tobacco control programmes, these costs can be overwhelmingly offset by raising tobacco taxes – which themselves are highly effective at reducing tobacco use. Recent progress has highlighted the feasibility of achieving smoke-free environments and generated increased worldwide interest in promoting them.

This report documents many gains in tobacco control achieved over the past year. Nearly 400 million people are newly covered by at least one complete MPOWER measure because of the actions taken by 17 countries to fight the tobacco epidemic. Of particular note is the progress made

on establishing smoke-free environments, which is the focus of the report.

Seven countries, most of which are middle-income, newly adopted comprehensive smoke-free laws in 2008. Several of these countries progressed from having either no national smoke-free law or only minimal protection in some types of public places or workplaces to full protection in all types of places. However, the data presented here also show that we have much more to do. Despite progress, only 9% of countries mandate smoke-free bars and restaurants, and 65 countries report no implementation of any smoke-free policies on a national level.

The WHO Framework Convention on Tobacco Control sets the bar high and establishes strong momentum for moving forward with global tobacco control. As documented in this report, progress is being made – but we can and must do more. Governments around the world, in partnership with civil society, must continue to act decisively against the tobacco epidemic – the leading global cause of preventable death. By continuing to make tobacco control a top priority, we can build on our successes and create a tobacco-free world.

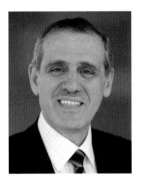

Dr Ala Alwan
Assistant Director-General
World Health Organization

Summary

Tobacco use is the leading cause of preventable death, and is estimated to kill more than 5 million people each year worldwide. Most of these deaths are in low- and middle-income countries. The gap in deaths between low- and middle-income countries and high-income countries is expected to widen further over the next several decades if we do nothing. If current trends persist, tobacco will kill more than 8 million people worldwide each year by the year 2030, with 80% of these premature deaths in low- and middle-income countries. By the end of this century, tobacco may kill a billion people or more unless urgent action is taken.

The success of the WHO FCTC, which as of July 2009 had more than 160 Parties covering 86% of the world's population, demonstrates the global political will for making tobacco control far more comprehensive and successful. The WHO Framework Convention and its guidelines provide the foundation for countries to implement and manage tobacco control. To help make this a reality, WHO introduced the MPOWER package of measures last year. The package is intended to assist in the country-level implementation of effective measures to reduce the demand for tobacco, contained in the WHO FCTC. As the Conference of the Parties carries out its work, MPOWER provides country-level practical assistance for those areas of the WHO FCTC that it covers. MPOWER focuses on demand measures, though WHO also recognizes the importance of and is committed to implementing the supply-side measures in the WHO FCTC.

In this year's *WHO Report on the Global Tobacco Epidemic, 2009*, all data on implementation of the six measures have been updated through 2008 and additional data have been collected on selected areas, as described in Technical Note I. Categories of policy achievement have been refined and, where possible, made consistent with new WHO FCTC guidelines. Last year's data have been reanalysed to be consistent with these new categories, allowing comparisons between 2007 and 2008. This year's printed report is presented in a more streamlined fashion; please see www.who.int/tobacco/mpower for all country-specific data.

This report provides a comprehensive overview of the evidence base for protecting people from the harms of second-hand tobacco smoke through legislation and enforcement. There is a special focus on the status of the implementation of smoke-free policies, with detailed data collected for the first time ever on a global basis at both the national level and for large subnational jurisdictions. Additional

154 million people, mostly in low- and middle-income countries, became newly covered by comprehensive smoke-free laws in 2008.

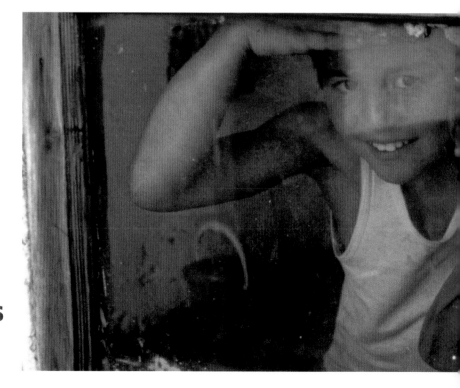

SHARE OF THE WORLD POPULATION COVERED BY SELECTED TOBACCO CONTROL POLICIES, 2008

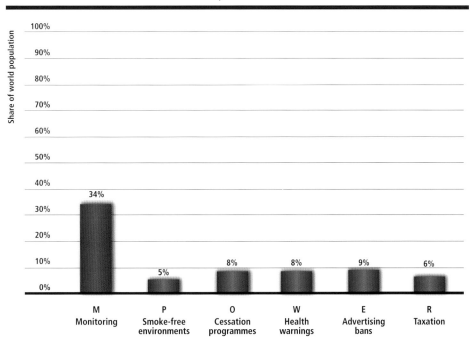

For the definitions of highest categories depicted here, please refer to Technical Note I.

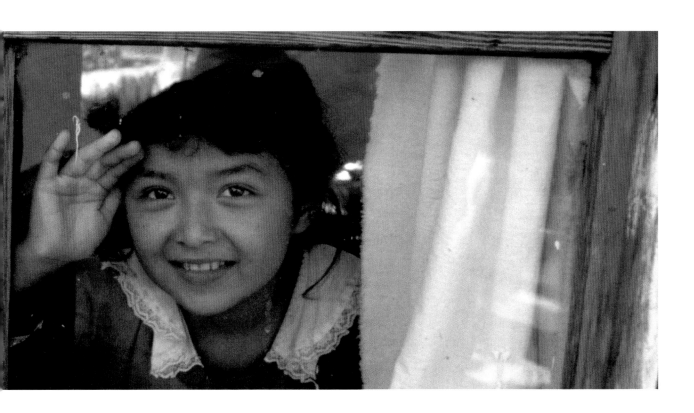

analyses of smoke-free legislation were performed, allowing for a more detailed understanding of progress and future challenges in this area.

Although progress in implementing the MPOWER measures has been made, with nearly 400 million people newly covered by at least one complete measure during 2008, there is still considerable work to be done. Less than 10% of the world's population is covered by any one of the measures.

The report's focus on smoke-free legislation shows that much more progress is needed in this area. In 2008, 154 million people, mostly in middle-income countries, became newly covered by comprehensive smoke-free laws. Smoke-free policies at the subnational level are becoming increasingly common, and progress at the subnational level should continue and be encouraged alongside national progress. Of the 100 biggest

cities in the world, only 22 are completely smoke-free but progress continues – since completion of data collection for this report, three additional large cities in Brazil (Rio de Janeiro, Salvador and São Paulo) have passed comprehensive smoke-free legislation*. Cities and other subnational jurisdictions can protect their citizens even before national legislation is in place. Despite these positive signs, more than 90% of the world's population is not protected by comprehensive smoke-free policies. Further, compliance with smoke-free laws is low: only 2% of the world's population live in countries with comprehensive smoke-free laws and high levels of compliance with these laws.

Alarmingly, progress on advertising and marketing bans has stalled, with virtually no progress in 2008. Only Panama passed a new advertising ban, leaving more than 91% of the world's population without the protection afforded by a comprehensive advertising ban. Progress on increasing

taxes is too slow – although some countries have made progress, others have slid backwards. Nearly 94% of the world's population live in a country where taxes represent less than 75% of the cigarette pack price. Increasing taxes during this time of financial hardship is universally beneficial – governments can increase their revenues, and smoking prevalence can be greatly reduced. Even with existing tax rates, tobacco control remains severely under-funded. Globally, more than 170 times as many dollars are collected through annual tobacco tax revenues as are spent each year on tobacco control.

* Please refer to Table 2.4.0 for detailed information.

There is still considerable work to be done. Less than 10% of the world's population is covered by any one of the MPOWER measures.

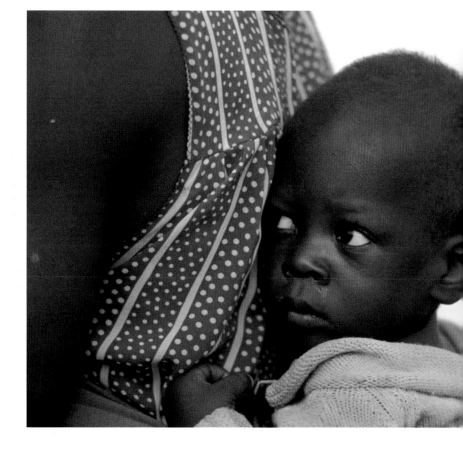

THE STATE OF SELECTED TOBACCO CONTROL POLICIES IN THE WORLD, 2008

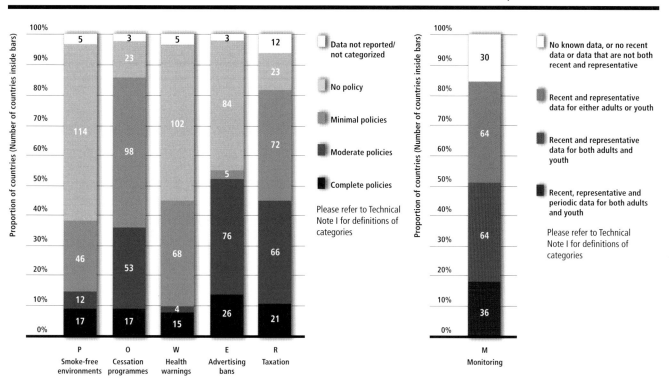

Left chart — Proportion of countries (Number of countries inside bars)

	P Smoke-free environments	O Cessation programmes	W Health warnings	E Advertising bans	R Taxation
Data not reported/not categorized	5	3	5	3	12
No policy	114	23	102	84	23
Minimal policies	46	98	68	5	72
Moderate policies	12	53	4	76	66
Complete policies	17	17	15	26	21

Legend:
- Data not reported/not categorized
- No policy
- Minimal policies
- Moderate policies
- Complete policies

Please refer to Technical Note I for definitions of categories

Right chart — Proportion of countries (Number of countries inside bars)

	M Monitoring
No known data	30
Recent and representative data for either adults or youth	64
Recent and representative data for both adults and youth	64
Recent, representative and periodic data for both adults and youth	36

Legend:
- No known data, or no recent data or data that are not both recent and representative
- Recent and representative data for either adults or youth
- Recent and representative data for both adults and youth
- Recent, representative and periodic data for both adults and youth

Please refer to Technical Note I for definitions of categories

INCREASE IN THE SHARE OF THE WORLD POPULATION COVERED BY SELECTED TOBACCO CONTROL POLICIES SINCE 2007

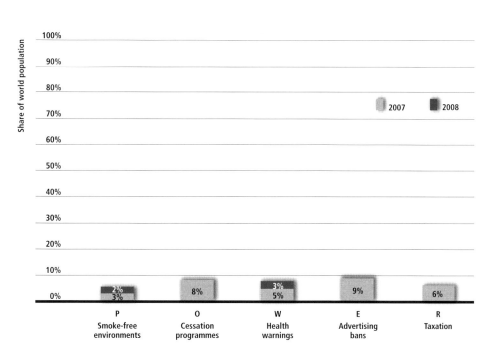

2007 / 2008

	P Smoke-free environments	O Cessation programmes	W Health warnings	E Advertising bans	R Taxation
2007	2%	8%	3%	9%	6%
2008	3%	8%	5%	9%	6%

Notes: Changes of at least 1% are shown in this graph.
   Data on monitoring are not shown in this graph because they are not comparable between 2007 and 2008.

WHO Framework Convention on Tobacco Control

The WHO Framework Convention on Tobacco Control (WHO FCTC), developed in response to the globalization of the tobacco epidemic, is the first treaty negotiated by the Member States of the World Health Organization using their powers under the Organization's Constitution. It is the pre-eminent global tobacco control instrument, which contains legally binding obligations for its Parties, sets the baseline for reducing both demand for and supply of tobacco, and provides a comprehensive direction for tobacco control policy at all levels. The treaty's governing body, comprising all Parties, is the Conference of the Parties (COP), an intergovernmental entity that supervises the effective implementation of the treaty.

To address tobacco use's complex set of determinants, the WHO FCTC negotiators included both supply and demand reduction measures in the text. The core demand reduction provisions in the WHO FCTC are contained in Articles 6 and 8–14, entitled:

Article 6. Price and tax measures to reduce the demand for tobacco.

Article 8. Protection from exposure to tobacco smoke.
Article 9. Regulation of the contents of tobacco products.
Article 10. Regulation of tobacco product disclosures.
Article 11. Packaging and labelling of tobacco products.
Article 12. Education, communication, training and public awareness.
Article 13. Tobacco advertising, promotion and sponsorship.
Article 14. Reduction measures concerning tobacco dependence and cessation.

Scientific evidence has unequivocally established that exposure to tobacco smoke causes death, disease and disability.

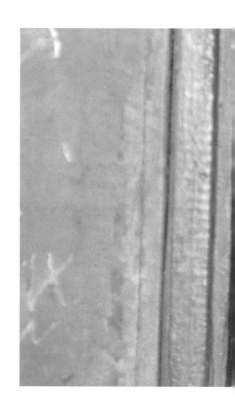

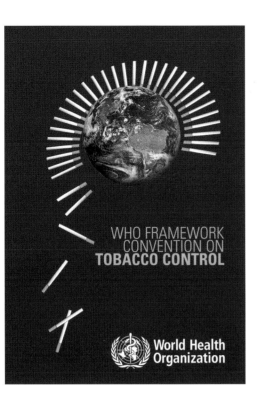

The core supply reduction provisions in the WHO FCTC are contained in Articles 15–17, entitled:

Article 15. Illicit trade in tobacco products.
Article 16. Sales to and by minors.
Article 17. Provision of support for economically viable alternative activities.

In adopting the WHO FCTC, the Member States of WHO:

- established the global standard for a concerted effort to fight the tobacco epidemic;
- reaffirmed the right of all people to the highest standard of health; and
- reinforced the role of international law in preventing disease and promoting health.

Since its entry into force on 27 February 2005, the WHO FCTC has become one of the most widely embraced treaties in the history of the United Nations, with more than 160 Parties, covering more than 86% of the world's population. The power of this treaty lies not only in its obligations, which are binding for all Parties, but also in the formal demonstration of the global commitment to take action against tobacco use – which kills millions of people and causes billions of dollars in economic damage every year.

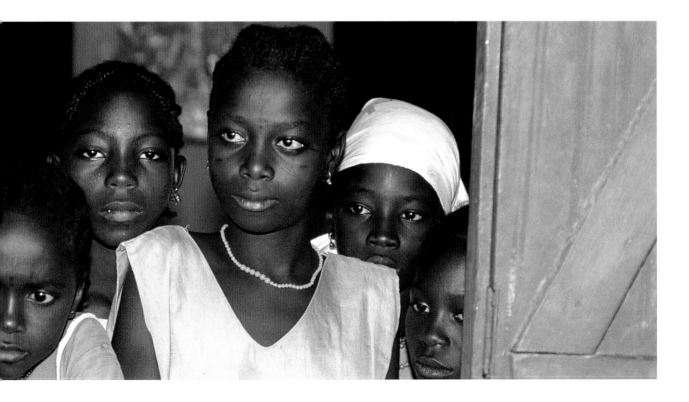

Article 8 – Protection from exposure to tobacco smoke

In developing the WHO FCTC, the overwhelming evidence of the beneficial effects of smoke-free places underpins Article 8 of the treaty (Protection from exposure to tobacco smoke), which includes the broad statement that "scientific evidence has unequivocally established that exposure to tobacco smoke causes death, disease and disability" (1). Article 8 forms the basis for international action to reduce the burden of disease attributable to second-hand tobacco smoke, and is especially important as it creates a legal obligation for the treaty's Parties to take action. The strength of the language and of the obligations set forth in Article 8 have led to measurable global improvements in protecting people from exposure to tobacco smoke, though there is still work to be done in most countries and in all regions.

Guidelines for the implementation of Article 8

The objectives of the Article 8 guidelines are "to assist Parties in meeting their obligations under Article 8 of the WHO Framework Convention on Tobacco Control, in a manner consistent with the scientific evidence regarding exposure to second-hand tobacco smoke and the best practice worldwide in the implementation of smoke free measures...[and] to identify the key elements of legislation necessary to effectively protect people from exposure to tobacco smoke, as required by Article 8" (2).

The Article 8 guidelines development process was a rapid and tangible success. During its second session in July 2007, the working group presented a completed set of draft guidelines for the implementation of Article 8, which the COP, representing all Parties to the WHO FCTC, adopted unanimously (2, 3).

The foundations of the COP guidelines are consistent with scientific evidence and well supported by best practices. The document establishes high standards of

There is no safe level of exposure to tobacco smoke. All people should be protected from such exposure.

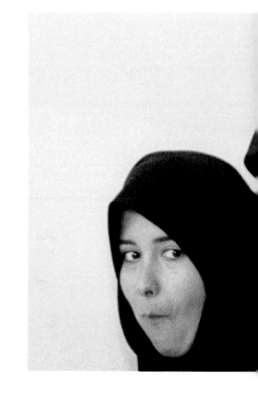

accountability for treaty compliance and includes principles and definitions of terms. The substance of the Article 8 guidelines is separated into four sections:

Scope of effective legislation

In this section, the guidelines state that Parties are obligated to pass measures that provide *universal* protection from tobacco smoke in all indoor public places, indoor workplaces, and public transport. Additionally, there are no legal or health justifications for exemptions. Each Party is expected to provide such protection within five years of entry into force of the treaty for that Party. The guidelines note that Article 8 also requires Parties to pass measures to protect people from exposure to tobacco smoke in "other" public places "as appropriate" (*3*). Parties are encouraged to consider the evidence of health

hazards and the protection that could be afforded to their populations when choosing these other places.

Inform, consult and involve the public to ensure support and smooth implementation

The critical issue of public awareness and support for smoke-free legislation is addressed in this section. The guidelines indicate that Parties should involve all stakeholders, in particular businesses that will be affected by smoke-free legislation, during the legislation development process. The association between high levels of public awareness and support and strong enforcement of smoke-free laws supports implementation of broad educational campaigns that include the following key messages:
1. the harm caused by second-hand tobacco smoke exposure;

2. the fact that elimination of indoor smoke is the only science-based solution to ensure complete protection from exposure;
3. the right of all workers to be equally protected by law; and
4. that smoke-free environments do not adversely affect economic interests, particularly those of the hospitality industry; rather, the evidence indicates economic benefits for all sectors in addition to any health benefits achieved.

Enforcement

The enforcement section indicates that Parties should adopt legislation that includes a duty of compliance by both businesses and smokers, with businesses required to take actions such as posting "no smoking" signs, removing all ashtrays, supervising observance of the rules and taking measures against individuals who break the rules. Penalties for failing to comply with this

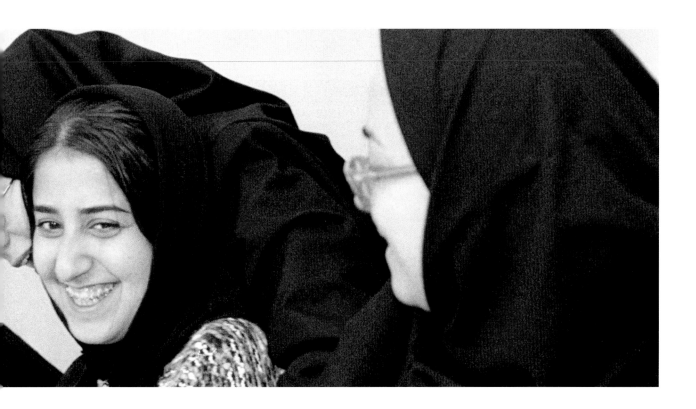

legislation should focus on businesses rather than individual smokers and should be large and/or serious enough to deter violations. Additionally, the authority responsible for enforcement should be identified within the enabling legislation, as should a system for monitoring compliance and prosecuting violators. Enforcement strategies include utilizing "soft enforcement" by warning violators immediately following passage of the legislation, transitioning into strong, decisive enforcement to ensure future compliance. Smoke-free laws often become self-enforcing over time; legislation should include an avenue for community members to report violations, as such reports can be one of the primary and most effective forms of enforcement.

Monitoring and evaluation of measures

Monitoring and evaluating the effects of the measures implemented in accordance with Article 8 are critical to maintain public awareness and support, study best practices and lessons learned, and identify the tobacco industry's efforts to undermine smoke-free policies. The guidelines provide eight key process and outcome indicators for monitoring and evaluation (3).

Perhaps most importantly, the COP guidelines for implementing Article 8 reiterate that there is no safe level of exposure to tobacco smoke, and that all people should be protected from such exposure. It is with these principles in mind that this report focuses on second-hand tobacco smoke and the protections from this health threat that the world's governments provide for their people.

WHO recommendations

In support of the development and drafting of the COP's Article 8 guidelines, WHO released detailed country-level policy recommendations for facilitating the passage and successful implementation and enforcement of smoke-free laws (4). Based on evidence of the cost-effectiveness, feasibility and popularity of smoke-free policies, and the successful experience of a rapidly growing number of jurisdictions worldwide, WHO makes the following four key policy recommendations to protect workers and the public from exposure to second-hand smoke (4):

1. Remove the source of the pollutant – tobacco smoke – by implementing 100% smoke-free environments. This is the only effective strategy to reduce exposure to second-hand tobacco smoke to safe levels in indoor environments and to provide an acceptable level of protection

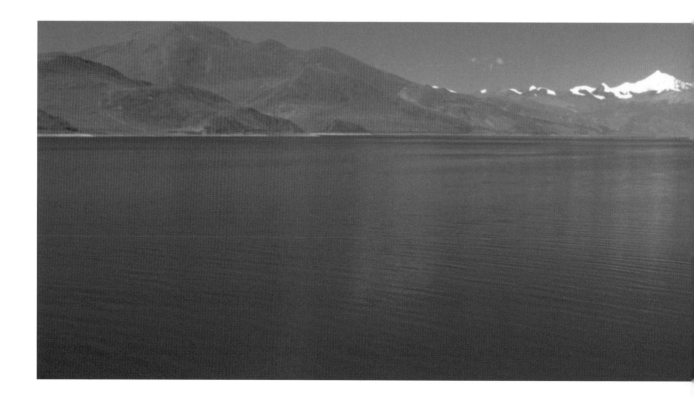

from the dangers of exposure. Ventilation and smoking areas, whether separately ventilated from non-smoking areas or not, do not reduce exposure to a safe level of risk and are not recommended.

2. Enact legislation requiring all indoor workplaces and public places to be 100% smoke-free environments. Laws should ensure universal and equal protection for all. Voluntary policies are not an acceptable response to protection. Under some circumstances, the principle of universal, effective protection may require specific quasi-outdoor and outdoor workplaces to be smoke-free.

3. Implement and enforce the law. Passing smoke-free legislation is not enough. Its proper implementation and adequate enforcement require relatively small but critical efforts and means.

4. Implement educational strategies to reduce second-hand tobacco smoke exposure in the home, recognizing that smoke-free workplace legislation increases the likelihood that people (both smokers and non-smokers) will voluntarily make their homes smoke-free.

Policy recommendations such as these are part of WHO's larger tobacco control programme driven by the WHO FCTC. To provide technical assistance to help Member States fulfil some of their commitments to the treaty, WHO has proposed the MPOWER package of measures. MPOWER supports the implementation of six effective tobacco control measures proven to reduce tobacco use: raising taxes and prices; banning advertising, promotion and sponsorship; protecting people from second-hand tobacco smoke; warning about the dangers of tobacco; offering help to people who want to quit; and carefully monitoring the epidemic and prevention policies (5). Each measure reflects one or more provisions of the WHO FCTC, and the package of six measures is an important entry point for scaling up efforts to reduce the demand for tobacco.

As part of MPOWER, WHO is developing practical training materials as well as assessment, surveillance and monitoring tools designed to support the WHO FCTC and its guidelines. MPOWER is an integral part of the WHO Action Plan for the Prevention and Control of Noncommunicable Diseases, which was endorsed at the 61st World Health Assembly in 2008 and reflects the commitment of WHO Member States to WHO FCTC implementation.

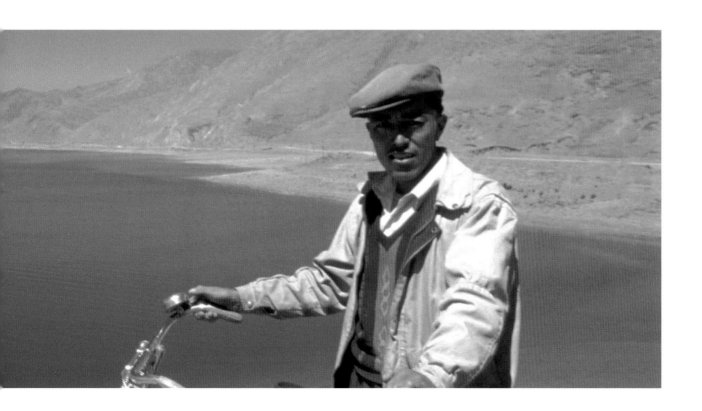

Protect people from tobacco smoke

Second-hand tobacco smoke is dangerous to health

Second-hand tobacco smoke is the smoke emitted from the burning end of a cigarette (side-stream smoke) or from other tobacco products, usually in combination with the mainstream smoke exhaled by the smoker, and has similar components to inhaled or mainstream smoke (6). However, it is three to four times more toxic per gram of particulate matter than mainstream tobacco smoke, and the toxicity of side-stream smoke is higher than the sum of the toxicities of its constituents (7).

More than 4 000 chemicals have been identified in tobacco smoke, at least 250 of which are known to be harmful and more than 50 of which are known to cause cancer (8, 9). People in places that allow smoking can be subject to significant levels of toxins, as pollution from tobacco smoke can reach levels that are much higher than levels of other environmental toxins, such as particles found in automobile exhaust. Studies have shown that pollution levels in indoor places that allow smoking are higher than levels found on busy roadways, in closed motor garages and during firestorms (10).

Second-hand tobacco smoke can spread from one room to another within a building, even if doors to the smoking area are closed. Toxic chemicals from second-hand tobacco smoke contamination persist well beyond the period of active smoking, and then cling to rugs, curtains, clothes, food, furniture and other materials. These toxins can remain in a room weeks and months after someone has smoked there (11, 12), even if windows are opened or fans or air filters are used. Filters can become a source for deposited chemicals that are then recycled back into the air of a room rather than removed. Tobacco toxins that build up over time, coating the surfaces of room elements and materials and smokers' belongings, are sometimes referred to as "third-hand smoke" (13).

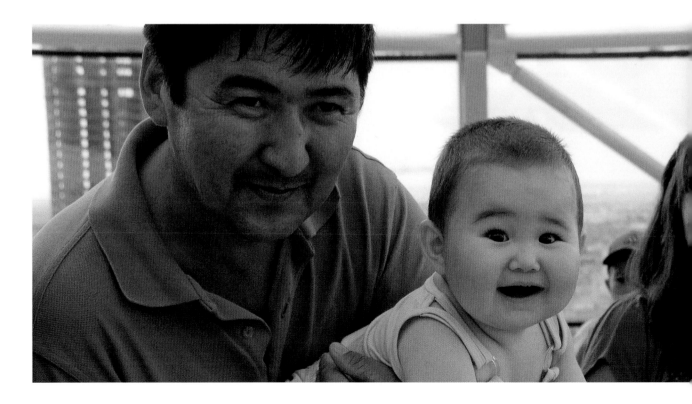

CHEMICALS CONTAINED IN SECOND-HAND TOBACCO SMOKE (PARTIAL LIST)

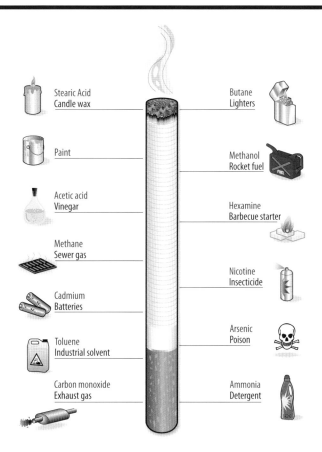

Stearic Acid
Candle wax

Paint

Acetic acid
Vinegar

Methane
Sewer gas

Cadmium
Batteries

Toluene
Industrial solvent

Carbon monoxide
Exhaust gas

Butane
Lighters

Methanol
Rocket fuel

Hexamine
Barbecue starter

Nicotine
Insecticide

Arsenic
Poison

Ammonia
Detergent

More than 4 000 chemicals have been identified in tobacco smoke.

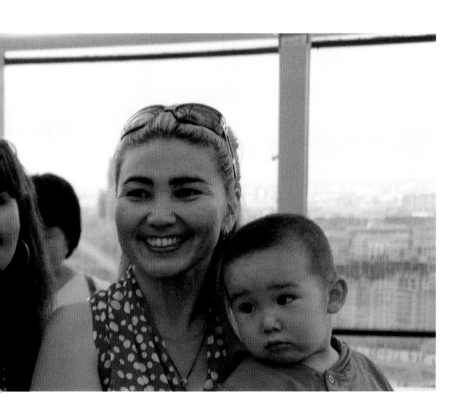

Exposure to second-hand tobacco smoke and early death

Second-hand tobacco smoke is present in virtually all public places where smoking is permitted (*14*), and there is no safe level of exposure (*15*).

Globally, it is estimated that about one third of adults are regularly exposed to second-hand tobacco smoke (*16*). In the European Union, 14% of non-smokers are exposed to other people's tobacco smoke at home, and a third of working adults are exposed to second-hand tobacco smoke at the workplace at least some of the time (*17*). In Canada, about a quarter of non-smokers report regular exposure at home, in vehicles or in public places (*18*).

An estimated 700 million children worldwide – about 40% of all children – are exposed to second-hand tobacco smoke at home (*19*). The global average of children with at least one smoking parent, according to the definition used by the Global Youth Tobacco Survey (GYTS), is estimated to be 43% (*20*). Data from the GYTS indicate that, among those surveyed, nearly half of youth aged 13 to 15 years who have never smoked are exposed to second-hand tobacco smoke at home, with a similar percentage exposed in places other than the home; these youth are 1.5 to 2 times more likely to initiate smoking than those not exposed (*20*).

Second-hand tobacco smoke is estimated to cause about 600 000 premature deaths per year worldwide (*16*), approximately the same number of people who are killed by measles or women who die during childbirth each year (*21*). Of all deaths attributable to second-hand tobacco smoke, 31% occur among children and 64% occur among women (*16*). About 50 000 deaths in the United States each year – about 11% of all tobacco-related deaths – are attributable to exposure to second-hand tobacco smoke (*22*). In the European Union, second-hand tobacco smoke exposure at work is estimated to cause about 7 600 deaths per year, with exposure at home causing an additional 72 100 deaths (*23*).

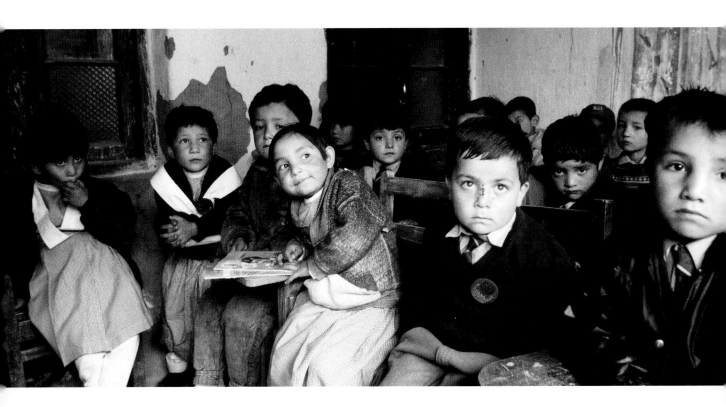

AVERAGE PERCENTAGE OF 13–15-YEAR-OLDS LIVING IN A HOME WHERE OTHERS SMOKE, BY WHO REGION, 2008

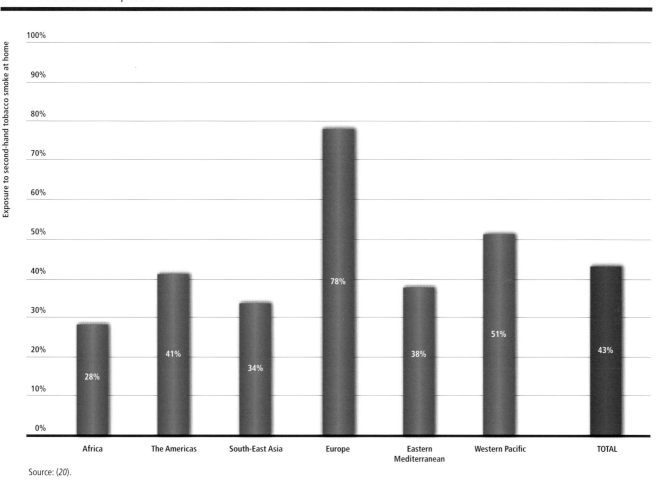

Exposure to second-hand tobacco smoke at home

Africa	The Americas	South-East Asia	Europe	Eastern Mediterranean	Western Pacific	TOTAL
28%	41%	34%	78%	38%	51%	43%

Source: (20).

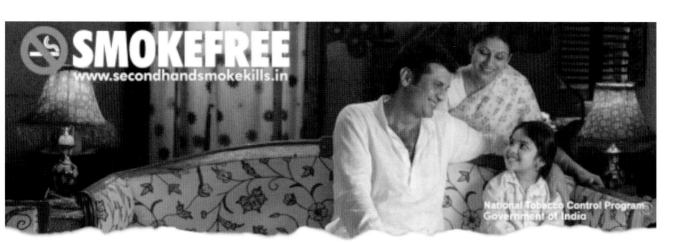

Globally, it is estimated that about one third of adults are regularly exposed to second-hand tobacco smoke.

Second-hand tobacco smoke exposure causes serious health problems

The scientific evidence of the health harms of smoking has been conclusively established for more than 50 years (24). However, smokers are not the only ones sickened and killed by tobacco: non-smokers who breathe air containing second-hand tobacco smoke also face increased risk of disease and death.

In the quarter century since evidence confirmed the health hazards of second-hand tobacco smoke (25–27), 14 scientific consensus reports by virtually all major medical and scientific organizations, including the WHO International Agency for Research on Cancer (6), the United States Surgeon General (28), the California Environmental Protection

Agency (29), and the United Kingdom Scientific Committee on Tobacco and Health (30) leave no doubt that exposure to second-hand tobacco smoke contributes to a range of serious and often fatal diseases in non-smokers.

Multiple studies confirm that exposure to second-hand tobacco smoke causes illness, disability and death from a wide range of diseases (31). Second-hand tobacco smoke exposure contributes to about 1% of the total global disease burden, and represents about 10–15% of the disease burden caused by active smoking (16). Second-hand tobacco smoke exposure is also associated with reduced health-related quality of life

among people who have never smoked, with higher levels of exposure resulting in a greater reduction in quality-of-life measures (32). Even house pets in homes where people smoke are more likely to develop cancer (33–35).

Among newborns exposed either in utero or after birth, there is an increased risk of premature birth (36) and low birth weight (37) and a doubling of the risk for Sudden Infant Death Syndrome (38). Among children exposed to second-hand tobacco smoke, there is a 50–100% higher risk of acute respiratory illness (39), higher incidence of ear infections (28) and an increased likelihood of developmental disabilities and behavioural problems (40, 41).

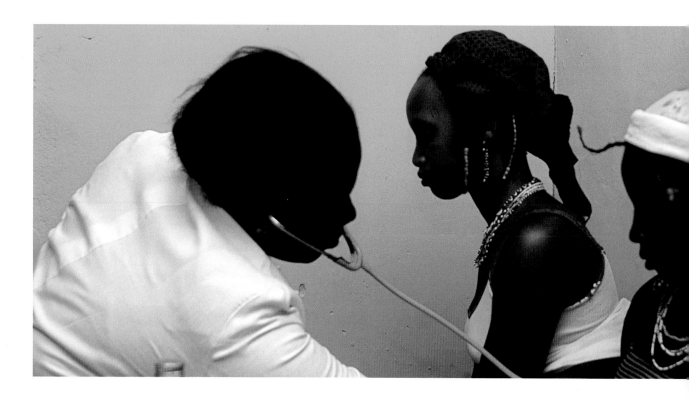

Breathing second-hand tobacco smoke has serious and often fatal health consequences.

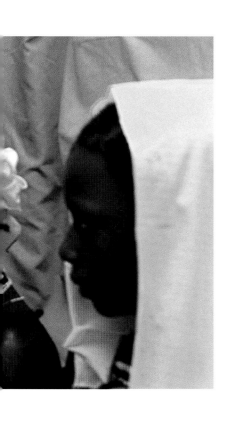

DISEASES CAUSED BY SECOND-HAND SMOKE

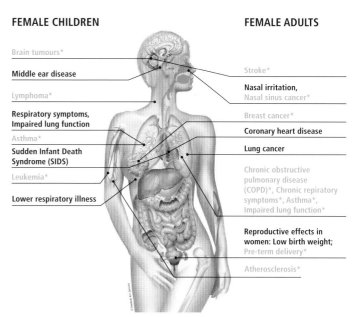

FEMALE CHILDREN

- Brain tumours*
- Middle ear disease
- Lymphoma*
- Respiratory symptoms, Impaired lung function
- Asthma*
- Sudden Infant Death Syndrome (SIDS)
- Leukemia*
- Lower respiratory illness

FEMALE ADULTS

- Stroke*
- Nasal irritation, Nasal sinus cancer*
- Breast cancer*
- Coronary heart disease
- Lung cancer
- Chronic obstructive pulmonary disease (COPD)*, Chronic repiratory symptoms*, Asthma*, Impaired lung function*
- Reproductive effects in women: Low birth weight; Pre-term delivery*
- Atherosclerosis*

* Evidence of causation: suggestive
Evidence of causation: sufficient

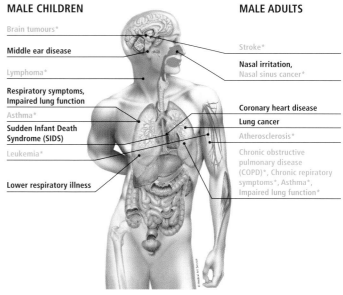

MALE CHILDREN

- Brain tumours*
- Middle ear disease
- Lymphoma*
- Respiratory symptoms, Impaired lung function
- Asthma*
- Sudden Infant Death Syndrome (SIDS)
- Leukemia*
- Lower respiratory illness

MALE ADULTS

- Stroke*
- Nasal irritation, Nasal sinus cancer*
- Coronary heart disease
- Lung cancer
- Atherosclerosis*
- Chronic obstructive pulmonary disease (COPD)*, Chronic repiratory symptoms*, Asthma*, Impaired lung function*

* Evidence of causation: suggestive
Evidence of causation: sufficient

Source: (28).

The economic threat of second-hand tobacco smoke

In addition to a large and growing health burden, second-hand tobacco smoke exposure also imposes economic burdens on individuals and countries, both for the costs of direct health care as well as indirect costs from reduced productivity. Second-hand tobacco smoke exposure in the United States alone costs an estimated US$ 5 billion annually in direct medical costs and another US$ 5 billion in indirect costs caused by productivity losses from lost wages due to disability and premature death (42). The US Occupational Health and Safety Administration estimated in 1994 that clean air increases productivity by 3% (43).

Several studies estimate that 10% of total tobacco-related economic costs are attributable to second-hand tobacco smoke exposure (44). The economic costs related to tobacco use in the United States total approximately US$ 193 billion per year (smoking-attributable health-care expenditures of US$ 96 billion and productivity losses of US$ 97 billion) (22).

Economic studies on the cost of tobacco use have been conducted in some other countries, but in most cases these do not assess costs specifically related to second-hand tobacco smoke exposure. Where data exist, economic costs related to second-hand tobacco smoke exposure elsewhere are roughly similar to those in the United States. In the China, Hong Kong Special Administrative Region, for example, the cost of direct medical care, long-term care and productivity losses attributable to second-hand tobacco smoke exposure is approximately US$ 156 million annually (about US$ 24 per capita, or 23% of total tobacco-related costs) (45).

COSTS OF TOBACCO-RELATED ILLNESS AND DEATH, CHINA, HONG KONG SPECIAL ADMINISTRATIVE REGION, 1998

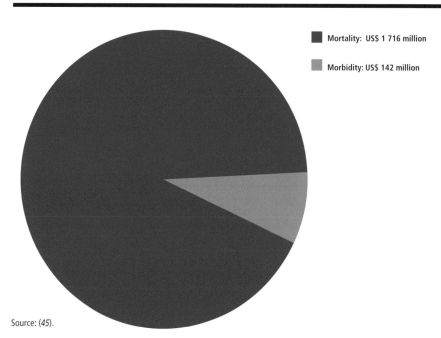

Mortality: US$ 1 716 million

Morbidity: US$ 142 million

Source: (45).

Smoke-free laws reduce exposure to second-hand tobacco smoke

The International Agency for Research on Cancer concluded: "there is sufficient evidence that implementation of smoke-free policies substantially decreases second-hand smoke exposure" (46). Studies of the effects of smoke-free policies consistently show that these policies decrease exposure to second-hand tobacco smoke by 80–90% in high-exposure settings, and that they can lead to overall decreases in exposure of up to 40% (47). People who work in places that are smoke-free are exposed to 3–8 times less second-hand tobacco smoke than other

workers (48). Non-smoking adults who live in communities with comprehensive smoke-free laws are 5–10 times less likely to be exposed to second-hand tobacco smoke than those who live where there is no smoke-free legislation (49). Ireland provides strong evidence of the effects of reducing exposure to second-hand tobacco smoke. Following the country's implementation of smoke-free legislation in 2004, ambient air nicotine and particulate matter concentrations in monitored indoor environments decreased by 83%, and there was a 79% reduction in exhaled breath

carbon monoxide and an 81% reduction in salivary cotinine* among bar workers. Bar workers' exposure to second-hand tobacco smoke plunged from 30 hours per week to zero (50, 51).

These findings were confirmed in numerous other places that enacted comprehensive smoke-free legislation. In Toronto, Canada, a complete smoke-free law for bars implemented in 2004 led to a reduction of 68% in the level of urinary cotinine* of bar workers in one month, while bar workers of a control community without

Smoke-free policies decrease exposure to second-hand tobacco smoke by 80–90% in high-exposure settings.

URINARY COTININE LEVELS AMONG BAR WORKERS IN TORONTO, CANADA, BEFORE AND AFTER INTRODUCTION OF COMPREHENSIVE SMOKE-FREE LEGISLATION

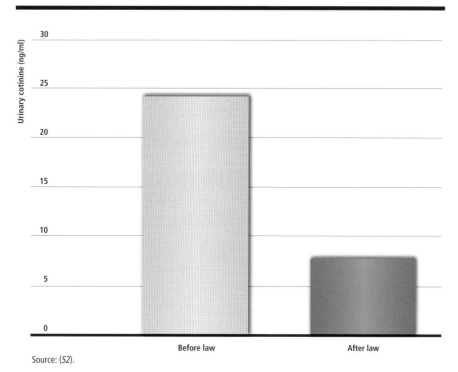

Source: (52).

* Analysis of salivary or urinary cotinine concentrations is used as a biological marker to measure exposure to second-hand tobacco smoke.

smoke-free legislation did not experience any significant change in the level of urinary cotinine levels (52). In Scotland, comprehensive smoke-free legislation enacted in 2006 resulted in an 86% decrease in the concentration of airborne particulate matter in pubs (53) and a 39% reduction in salivary cotinine levels among adult non-smokers (47).

In New York State, salivary cotinine levels in non-smoking adults decreased 47% in the year after enactment of a comprehensive smoking ban in 2003 (54); in New Zealand, comprehensive smoke-free legislation enacted in 2004 appears to have reduced exposure of bar patrons to second-hand tobacco smoke by about 90% (55); and in Finland, a nationally

implemented smoke-free law resulted in a reduction in second-hand tobacco smoke exposure in workplaces covered by this law, from 51% of workers reporting exposure before the law to 12% reporting exposure three years after the law became effective (56).

Enforcement needed to ensure protection against second-hand tobacco smoke

Based on the scientific evidence, the Conference of the Parties to the WHO Framework Convention of Tobacco Control (WHO FCTC) has concluded that 100% smoke-free environments are the only proven way to adequately protect the health of people from the harmful effects of second-hand tobacco smoke because no level of exposure is acceptable (2).

Once smoke-free laws have been enacted, governments must maintain strong

support through active and uniform enforcement that achieves high compliance levels, at least until such time as the law becomes self-enforcing. Although an increasing number of countries have passed legislation mandating smoke-free environments, the overwhelming majority of countries have no smoke-free laws, very limited laws, or ineffective enforcement. Legislation that is comprehensive, but that is not well enforced, does not protect against second-hand tobacco smoke

exposure, and legislation that covers only some places, even if well enforced, also does not provide significant protection.

Full enforcement of smoke-free laws is critical to establishing their credibility, especially immediately following their enactment (57). It may be necessary to actively and publicly enforce the law in the period directly after smoke-free laws are enacted to demonstrate the government's commitment to ensuring

100% smoke-free environments are the only proven way to adequately protect the health of people from the harmful effects of second-hand tobacco smoke.

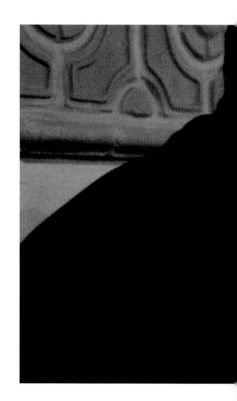

compliance. Unannounced inspections by the appropriate government agency can be very effective.

Once a high level of compliance is achieved, it may be feasible to reduce the level of formal enforcement, as maintenance of smoke-free places is largely self-enforcing in areas where the public and business communities support smoke-free policies

and legislation. Placing the responsibility for enforcing smoke-free places on facility owners and managers is the most effective way to ensure that the laws are enforced. In many countries, laws have established that business owners have a legal duty to provide safe workplaces for their employees. Levying of fines and other sanctions against business owners is more likely to ensure compliance than fining individual smokers.

Enforcement of legislation and its impact should be regularly monitored. Assessing and publicizing the lack of negative impact on business following enactment of smoke-free legislation will further enhance compliance with and acceptance of smoke-free laws.

Ventilation and designated smoking rooms are not effective

Smoking anywhere in a building significantly increases concentrations of second-hand tobacco smoke, even in parts of the building where people do not smoke (58). Physically separating smokers from non-smokers by allowing smoking only in designated smoking rooms reduces exposure to second-hand tobacco smoke only by about half, and thus provides only partial protection (59).

The American Society of Heating, Refrigerating and Air-Conditioning Engineers concluded in 2005 that comprehensive smoke-free laws are the only effective means of eliminating the risks associated with second-hand tobacco smoke, and that ventilation techniques should not be relied upon to control health risks from second-hand tobacco smoke

exposure (60, 61). This position statement concurs with other findings that ventilation and designated smoking rooms do not prevent exposure to second-hand tobacco smoke (62, 63).

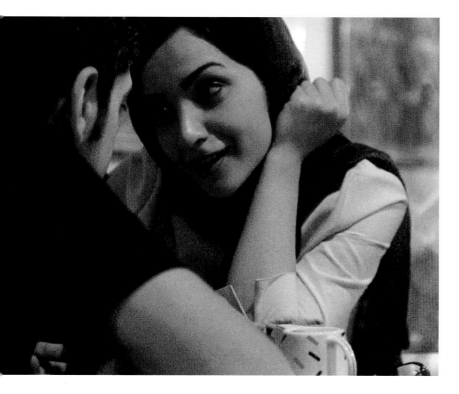

Ventilation and designated smoking rooms do not prevent exposure to second-hand tobacco smoke.

Health impact of smoke-free regulations

Smoke-free laws reduce respiratory symptoms

Because of the immediate drop in pollution levels and second-hand tobacco smoke exposure after implementation of smoke-free laws (*64*), improvements in respiratory health are experienced very quickly. In Scotland, bar workers reported a 26% decrease in respiratory symptoms, and asthmatic bar workers had reduced airway inflammation within three months after comprehensive smoke-free legislation was enacted (*65*). In California, bartenders reported a 59% reduction in respiratory symptoms and a 78% reduction in sensory irritation symptoms within eight weeks after implementation of the law requiring bars to be smoke-free (*66*).

Smoke-free laws reduce illness from heart disease

Even low-level exposure to second-hand tobacco smoke has a clinically significant effect on cardiovascular disease risk (*67*). Smoke-free environments reduce the incidence of heart attack among the general population almost immediately, even in the first few months after being implemented (*68*). Several studies have confirmed decreases in hospital admissions for heart attacks after comprehensive smoke-free legislation was enacted (*69–74*). Moreover, many of these studies, conducted in subnational areas (states/ provinces and cities) where smoke-free laws had not been enacted on a national level, show not only the impact of such laws, but also the potential benefit of enacting smoke-free legislation on a local level when national bans are not in place.

Smoke-free laws are expected to reduce lung cancer

Because of the long time lag between second-hand smoke exposure and the development of lung cancer, complete data are not yet available regarding the expected decline in lung cancer after implementation of smoke-free policies. Between 1988 and 2004, a period during which the state of California implemented comprehensive smoke-free legislation, rates of lung and bronchial cancer declined four times faster in California than in the rest of the United States, although at least some of this decrease may result from the sharper decline in smoking prevalence experienced in California compared with the rest of the country that began in the early 1980s (*75*).

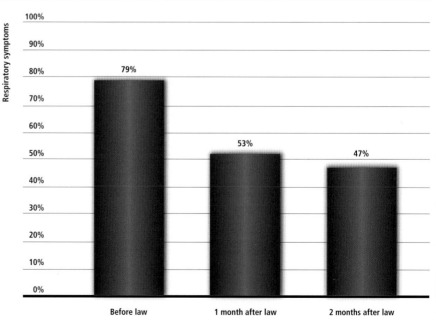

RESPIRATORY SYMPTOMS OF BAR WORKERS IN SCOTLAND, BEFORE AND AFTER INTRODUCTION OF COMPREHENSIVE SMOKE-FREE LEGISLATION

Source: (*65*).

Other benefits of smoke-free regulations

Smoke-free laws help smokers to reduce smoking or quit

Smoke-free environments not only protect non-smokers, they reduce tobacco use in continuing smokers by 2–4 cigarettes a day (76) and help smokers who want to quit, as well as former smokers who have already stopped, to quit successfully over the long term. Per capita cigarette consumption in the United States is between 5% and 20% lower in states with comprehensive smoke-free laws than in states without such laws (77).

Complete workplace smoking bans implemented in several industrialized nations are estimated to have reduced smoking prevalence among workers by an average of 3.8%, reduced average tobacco consumption by 3.1 cigarettes per day among workers who continue to smoke, and reduced total tobacco consumption among workers by an average of 29% (78). People who work in environments with smoke-free policies are nearly twice as likely to quit smoking as those in worksites without such policies, and people who continue to smoke decrease their average daily consumption by nearly four cigarettes per day (79).

After comprehensive smoke-free legislation was enacted in Ireland, about 46% of smokers reported that the law had made them more likely to quit; among those who did quit, 80% reported that the law had helped them to quit and 88% reported

Smoke-free environments not only protect non-smokers, they reduce tobacco use in continuing smokers and help smokers who want to quit.

EFFECTS OF IRELAND'S SMOKE-FREE LAW ON SMOKERS' REPORTED BEHAVIOURS

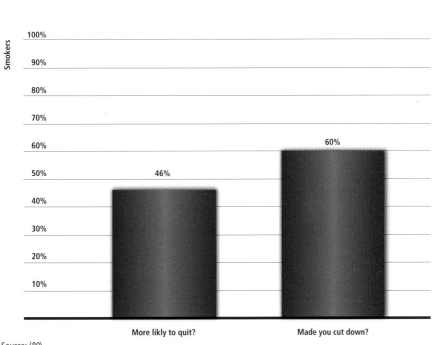

Source: (80).

that the law helped them to maintain cessation (80). In Scotland, 44% of people who quit smoking said that smoke-free legislation had helped them to quit (81).

Smoke-free laws encourage establishment of smoke-free homes

Legislation mandating smoke-free public places also encourages families to make their homes smoke-free (82), which protects children and other family members from exposure to second-hand tobacco smoke (83). In Australia, the introduction of smoke-free workplace laws in the 1990s was accompanied by a steep increase in the proportion of adults who avoided exposing children to second-hand tobacco smoke in the home (84). Even smokers are likely to voluntarily implement a "no smoking" rule in their homes after comprehensive smoke-free legislation is enacted (85, 86).

Voluntary smoke-free home policies also decrease adult and youth smoking. Home smoking bans reduce progression to smoking experimentation among youths who live with non-smokers. Teenagers who live in homes where smoking is allowed are nearly twice as likely to start smoking, even if adults are non-smokers themselves, than in homes where smoking is prohibited (87).

Smoke-free laws are popular

Public opinion surveys show that smoke-free legislation is extremely popular wherever it is enacted, even among smokers, and that support tends to increase over time after these laws are in place. Support is generally strongest for making hospitals and other health-care facilities smoke-free, while there is usually the least support for making bars and pubs smoke-free (88–90).

In 2006, Uruguay became the first country in the Americas to become 100% smoke-free by enacting a ban on smoking in all public spaces and workplaces, including bars, restaurants and casinos. The law won support from eight out of every 10 Uruguayans, including nearly two thirds of the country's smokers (91). After New Zealand passed smoke-free laws in 2004, 69% of its citizens said they supported the right of people to work in a smoke-free environment (92).

The smoke-free workplace law introduced in Ireland in March 2004 has been judged successful by 96% of people, including 89% of smokers (93). In California, 75% of the population approved of smoke-free workplace laws that included restaurants

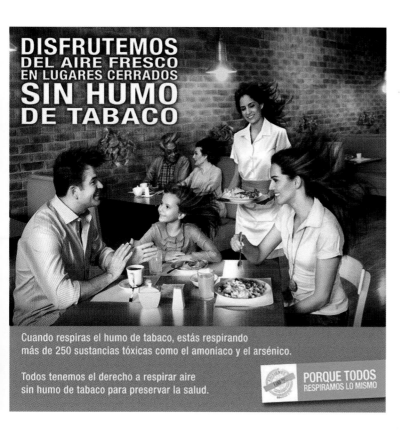

DISFRUTEMOS DEL AIRE FRESCO EN LUGARES CERRADOS SIN HUMO DE TABACO

Cuando respiras el humo de tabaco, estás respirando más de 250 sustancias tóxicas como el amoníaco y el arsénico.

Todos tenemos el derecho a respirar aire sin humo de tabaco para preservar la salud.

PORQUE TODOS RESPIRAMOS LO MISMO

In every country where comprehensive smoke-free legislation has been enacted, smoke-free environments are popular and result in either a neutral or positive impact on business.

and bars within the first few years after being enacted by that state in 1998 (*94*).

Although China has few smoke-free public places, 90% of people living in large cities – smokers and non-smokers alike – support a ban on smoking on public transport and in schools and hospitals (*95*). More than 80% of urban residents in China support smoke-free legislation in workplaces, and about half support banning smoking in restaurants and bars (*95*). In Russia, which also has few restrictions on smoking in public places, nearly a third of people support a complete ban on smoking in restaurants (*96*).

Smoke-free laws do not hurt business

Despite tobacco and hospitality industry claims, experience shows that in every country where comprehensive smoke-free legislation has been enacted, smoke-free environments are popular, easy to implement and enforce, and result in either a neutral or positive impact on businesses, including the hospitality sector (*97, 98*). These findings were similar in all places studied, including in Australia, Canada, the United Kingdom and the United States (*99*); Norway (*100*); New Zealand (*101*); the state of California (*102*); New York City (*103*); and various US states and municipalities (*104*).

In New York City, which implemented smoke-free legislation in two stages (covering most workplaces including most restaurants in 1995 and adding bars and remaining restaurants in 2003), restaurant employment increased after enactment of the 1995 law (*105*). Combined bar and restaurant employment and receipts increased in the year after enactment of the 2003 ordinance (*103*), and have continued increasing since.

After comprehensive smoke-free legislation was implemented, there were no statistically significant changes observed among hospitality industry economic indicators in Massachusetts (*106*), no economic harm to bar and restaurant businesses reported in the mid-sized US city of Lexington, Kentucky (*107*), and no adverse economic impact on tourism in Florida (*108*). When bars located in communities with smoke-free laws were sold, they commanded prices comparable to prices paid for similar bars in areas with no restrictions on smoking (*109*). This type of economic evidence can be used to counter false tobacco industry claims that establishing smoke-free places causes economic harm (*97, 110*).

AVERAGE ANNUAL EMPLOYMENT IN NEW YORK CITY RESTAURANTS AND BARS, BEFORE AND AFTER COMPREHENSIVE SMOKE-FREE LEGISLATION

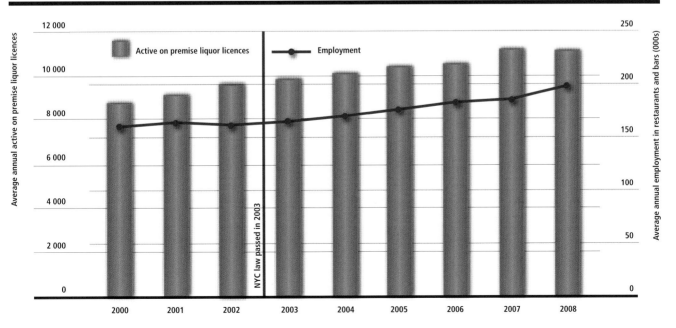

Source: (*103*) and additional unpublished data from the New York State Liquor Authority and New York City Economic Development Corporation.
Note: Average annual employment calculated from monthly totals.

Tobacco industry efforts to avoid 100% smoke-free legislation

The tobacco industry has long known that side-stream second-hand tobacco smoke contains higher concentrations of carcinogenic substances than does mainstream tobacco smoke (7). In a confidential 1978 report, the industry described increasing public concerns about second-hand tobacco smoke exposure as "the most dangerous development to the viability of the tobacco industry that has yet occurred" (111). The industry acknowledges the effectiveness of smoke-free environments, and how creating exceptions can undermine their impact. A 1992 internal report by Philip Morris stated: "Total prohibition of smoking in the workplace strongly affects industry volume. … Milder workplace restrictions, such as smoking only in designated areas, have much less impact on quitting rates and very little effect on consumption" (112).

The tobacco industry has a history of creating the appearance of scientific controversy in an attempt to counter initiatives intended to restrict tobacco use. However, the ultimate goal of these types of industry-backed initiatives is to maintain the social acceptability of smoking and prevent adoption of meaningful smoke-free policies in public places and in workplaces (113). Measures such as ventilation and separate smoking rooms, promoted as "reasonable" accommodations by the tobacco industry, also undermine the intended effects of legislative measures by continuing to expose people to second-hand tobacco smoke and reducing the incentive for smokers to quit (114).

Despite the incontrovertible scientific evidence of the harms of second-hand tobacco smoke, the tobacco industry has referred to such findings as "junk science" in an attempt to discredit them (115). The industry has also used front groups in an attempt to successfully convince some people to resist accepting these findings. Much of the impetus for discrediting scientific studies of the health effects of second-hand tobacco smoke comes from the tobacco industry, which develops and publicizes its own biased research to minimize the harmful effects of second-hand tobacco smoke because it fears that restrictions on smoking will reduce sales and profits (116–119). The tobacco industry has also resorted to attacks on researchers studying the effects of second-hand tobacco smoke by criticizing their motives or qualifications, even while acknowledging internally the validity of their research findings (120, 121).

Researchers funded by or affiliated with the tobacco industry are nearly 100 times more likely than independent researchers to conclude that second-hand tobacco smoke is not harmful to health (122). Much of the research funded by the tobacco industry is not published in peer-reviewed medical journals, is of poor scientific quality, and should not be used in scientific, legal or policy settings unless its quality has been independently assessed (123). The tobacco industry has even attempted to create its own peer-reviewed medical journals to publish papers on the effects of second-hand tobacco smoke that are favourable to its interests (124). A US federal court has ruled that tobacco industry assertions that second-hand tobacco smoke exposure does not cause disease are "fraudulent" (125).

The tobacco industry has a history of creating the appearance of scientific controversy in an attempt to counter initiatives intended to restrict tobacco use.

Key recommendations

These key recommendations – consistent with the WHO FCTC Article 8 guidelines – build on lessons learned from the experiences of several countries and hundreds of subnational and local jurisdictions that have successfully implemented laws requiring indoor workplaces and public places to be 100% smoke-free, as follows (*4*):

1. Legislation that mandates completely smoke-free environments – not voluntary policies – is necessary to protect public health.

2. Legislation should be simple, clear and enforceable, and comprehensive.

3. Action should be taken at any and all jurisdictional level(s) where effective legislation can be achieved.

4. Anticipating and responding to the tobacco industry's opposition, often mobilized through third parties, is crucial.

5. Involving civil society is central to achieving effective legislation.

6. Education and consultation with stakeholders are necessary to ensure smooth implementation.

7. An implementation and enforcement plan together with an infrastructure for enforcement, including high-profile prosecutions to include fines or closing of businesses of repeat violators, are critical for successful implementation.

8. Monitoring of implementation and compliance is essential, as is measurement of the impact of smoke-free environments; ideally, experiences should also be documented and the results made available to other jurisdictions to support their efforts to successfully introduce and implement effective legislation.

9. Physically separating smokers from non-smokers (for example by establishing designated smoking rooms) or providing ventilation of smoking areas does not eliminate the health risk resulting from exposure to second-hand tobacco smoke.

Because smokers and non-smokers alike are vulnerable to the harmful health effects of second-hand tobacco smoke, governments are obligated to protect health as a fundamental human right (*3*). This duty is implicit in the right to life and the right to the highest attainable standard of health as recognized in many international legal instruments, including the International Covenant on Economic, Social and Cultural Rights; the Convention on the Elimination of All Forms of Discrimination against Women; and the Convention on the Rights of the Child. These are formally incorporated into the Preamble of the WHO FCTC, and have been ratified in the constitutions of more than 100 countries. Voluntary agreements, often promoted by the tobacco industry as a "compromise", have proven insufficient to achieve public health goals because they do not eliminate, and at best only reduce, exposure to second-hand tobacco smoke (*126*). Comprehensive smoke-free legislation with strong enforcement is the best strategy for reducing exposure to second-hand tobacco smoke.

Recent progress has highlighted the feasibility of achieving smoke-free environments and generated increased worldwide interest in promoting them. Although much more work remains to be done, there are many examples where there have been improvements in smoke-free policies. Even smoking bans in restaurants, bars and other hospitality venues, generally considered the most difficult places to make smoke-free, have been successfully implemented in several countries with near universal compliance and strong public support. Other countries can learn from these experiences as they create and expand smoke-free environments for the vast majority of people worldwide who remain without protection against the harm of second-hand tobacco smoke exposure.

There is no risk-free level of exposure to tobacco smoke. The health risk resulting from exposure to second-hand tobacco smoke is the primary reason to ban smoking in workplaces and public places, because an individual's decision to smoke results in damage to others. Smoke-free environments help guarantee the right of non-smokers to breathe clean air, motivate smokers to quit, and allow governments to take the lead in tobacco prevention through highly popular health measures.

Implementation of effective measures is gaining momentum

mpower **Monitor tobacco use and prevention policies**

Monitoring needs to be representative and repeated regularly

Surveillance, monitoring and evaluation form the cornerstone of well-informed tobacco control policy development. A number of articles in the WHO FCTC require data collection, but Article 20 (*Research, surveillance and exchange of information*) and Article 21 (*Reporting and exchange of information*) elaborate the broad surveillance requirements that are the foundation for implementation of monitoring.

Surveillance, monitoring and evaluation systems must use standardized and scientifically valid data collection and analysis practices. Population surveys using a representative, randomly selected sample of sufficiently large size can provide the needed estimates, and can be conducted on tobacco use alone or combined with surveys of other priority health issues of interest to a country's health ministry. Such surveys should be repeated at regular intervals using the same questions, sampling, data analysis and reporting techniques. Comparable data across different survey periods are required to accurately monitor and evaluate the

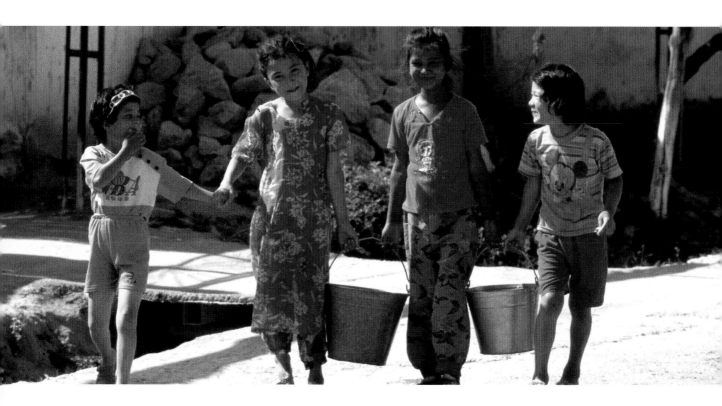

MONITORING

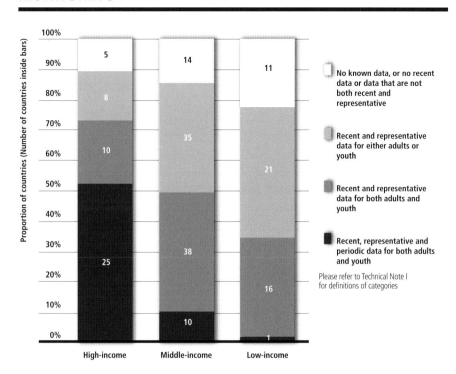

- No known data, or no recent data or data that are not both recent and representative
- Recent and representative data for either adults or youth
- Recent and representative data for both adults and youth
- Recent, representative and periodic data for both adults and youth

Please refer to Technical Note I for definitions of categories

Monitoring activities can provide critical evidence to bolster the case for stronger tobacco control.

MONITOR THE PREVALENCE OF TOBACCO USE – HIGHEST ACHIEVING COUNTRIES, 2008

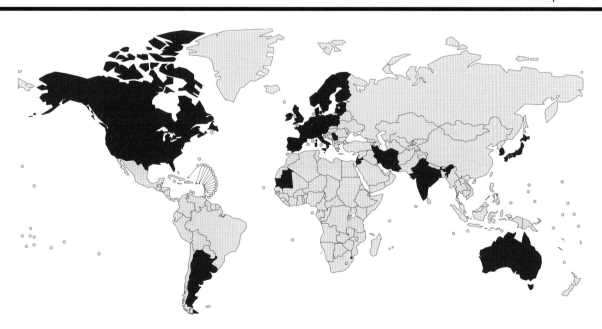

impact of tobacco control interventions over time. Standardized questions about tobacco use can be embedded in existing population-based surveys or censuses.

Other monitoring activities that should be undertaken include assessments of government enforcement of and societal compliance with tobacco control policies, including tax collection and tax evasion, smoke-free places, and advertising and marketing bans.

The extent and type of tobacco advertising, marketing and promotional activities, including tobacco industry sponsorship of public and private events, should also be monitored. The importance of eliminating tobacco industry interference in tobacco control efforts is recognized by WHO FCTC Article 5.3, which requires Parties to "act to protect [their public health] policies from commercial and other vested interests of the tobacco industry". Understanding that this provision is a keystone to effective tobacco control, the Conference of the Parties adopted guidelines on its implementation by consensus in November 2008 (3).

Monitoring activities can provide critical evidence to bolster the case for stronger tobacco control policies, and should be widely disseminated to enable governments, country leadership, and civil society to use them to develop tobacco control policies and build capacity for effective implementation and enforcement of the other MPOWER interventions.

Only one third of countries have recent, representative and periodically repeated data from monitoring systems

■ Overall, monitoring activities are strongest in high-income countries. Progress is particularly needed in low- and middle-income countries, where tobacco use is rising fastest.
■ More than 20% of low-income countries and about 15% of middle-income countries have no national smoking prevalence data for adults or youth, or data that are not recent and/ or representative.

■ A total of 100 countries, with 55% of the world's population (compared with 48% in 2007), have recent and representative data on smoking prevalence for both adults and youth from surveys conducted in 2003 or later. However, only 36 countries, with 34% of the world's population, also collect data on a periodic basis (i.e. at intervals of five years or less).

Surveillance, monitoring and evaluation form the cornerstone of well-informed tobacco control policy development.

Turkey expands tobacco use surveys

Data on smoking prevalence and patterns of tobacco use among adults and youth that are both recent and representative of the national population are key to successful guidance of tobacco control programmes. Turkey has shown a commitment to surveillance, beginning with its first implementation of the Global Youth Tobacco Survey (GYTS) on a nationally and regionally representative sample of students aged 13–15 years in 2003, and with the 2003 implementation of WHO's World Health Survey.

In 2009, Turkey repeated the GYTS with nationally and regionally representative samples of four regions within the country (the three largest cities – Ankara, Istanbul and Izmir – and the rest of the country). This representative sample design will allow for direct comparisons between the 2003 and 2009 data to show progress and challenges in Turkey's tobacco control efforts.

In December 2008, Turkey was the first country to complete data collection for the Global Adult Tobacco Survey (GATS), a survey instrument launched as a new component of CDC/WHO's Global Tobacco Surveillance System. GATS was introduced in 14 low- and middle-income countries with large numbers of smokers. GATS is a standardized household adult tobacco survey that collects data among adults aged 15 years or older on smoking prevalence and patterns; exposure to second-hand tobacco smoke; cessation attempts; exposure to media; and knowledge, attitude and perceptions of the harm caused by tobacco use and of tobacco control measures.

Results from GATS in Turkey show that 31% of adults aged 15 years and older (48% of males and 15% of females) are current smokers. Tobacco use is most prevalent among people aged 25–44 years, with 40% this age group reporting current smoking. More than half of Turkey's adults have never smoked, and 95% of adults are aware of health warnings on cigarette packages.

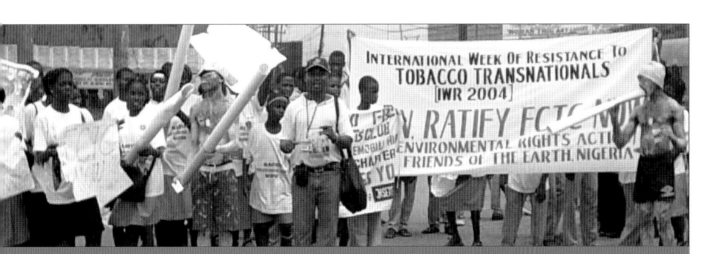

Monitoring tobacco industry activities in Nigeria

In addition to collecting data on smoking prevalence and other measures of tobacco use, it is also necessary to monitor the activities of the tobacco industry. In Africa, the industry has in recent years greatly increased its presence and engaged in aggressive marketing campaigns, targeting youth in particular.

In Nigeria, one nongovernmental organization, Environmental Rights Action/Friends of the Earth (Nigeria ERA/FOTEN) has successfully identified front groups created and used by the tobacco industry to help carry out its activities. It has highlighted the industry's unfair practices towards tobacco farmers and indifference to the use of child labour, revealed the existence of industry-sponsored music concerts and other events that appeal to youth where cigarettes and tobacco-related merchandise have been distributed freely, and uncovered industry cooperation programmes with various government institutions and corporate social responsibility initiatives.

ERA/FOTE has also greatly strengthened the capacity of many smaller organizations to become engaged in industry monitoring and grassroots advocacy, and is spearheading formation of the Nigeria Tobacco Control Alliance, a coalition of nongovernmental organizations active in the fight against tobacco.

Protect from tobacco smoke

Progress in implementing smoke-free policies

There was notable progress between 2007 and 2008 in protecting people from the harms of second-hand tobacco smoke. Seven more countries (Colombia, Djibouti, Guatemala, Mauritius, Panama, Turkey and Zambia) joined the group of countries with complete policies in 2008, bringing the total number with comprehensive smoke-free laws to 17.

The total global population covered by comprehensive smoke-free laws increased from 3.1% to 5.4% in just one year, so that 154 million additional people worldwide are protected from the harms of second-hand tobacco smoke. Several of these countries progressed from having either no national smoke-free law or only minimal protection in some types of public places or workplaces to full protection in all types of places.

However, 114 countries at all levels of economic development still have the lowest level of legal protection: no smoke-free policies in place at all, or policies that cover only one or two of the eight types of public places assessed. Nearly half of high-income countries, and nearly two thirds of low- and middle-income countries, have the lowest level of protection. More than a third of high-income countries, about a quarter of middle-income and about a third of low-income countries have attained intermediate levels of achievement with three or more, but not all, types of public places and workplaces completely smoke-free.

The greatest progress in enacting comprehensive smoke-free laws was made among middle-income countries, with six out of seven additional countries that have enacted comprehensive policies covering all public places.

In several countries, in order to significantly expand the creation of smoke-free places including restaurants and bars, it was politically necessary to include exceptions to the law that allowed for the provision of designated smoking rooms. The requirements for designated smoking rooms are so technically complex and stringent that, for practical purposes, few or no establishments were expected to implement them. Because no data were requested on the number of complex designated smoking rooms actually constructed, it is not possible to know whether these laws have resulted in the complete absence of such rooms, as intended. For this reason, these few countries have not been categorized in the analyses for this section. Future data collection efforts will include such measures, as well as incorporate evaluation of legislation enforcement. As noted in the beginning of this report, as well as in the WHO FCTC Article 8 guidelines and multiple other governmental and nongovernmental reports, ventilation and

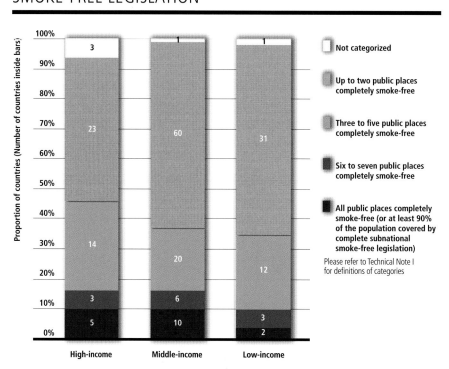

SMOKE-FREE LEGISLATION

other forms of designated smoking areas do not fully protect from the harms of second-hand tobacco smoke, and the only laws that provide complete protection are those that result in the complete absence of smoking in all public places.

Smoke-free legislation is more likely to cover some places than others

Only 17 countries currently have smoke-free policies that provide universal and effective protection from second-hand tobacco smoke. In the great majority of countries, workers and members of the public are not protected equally from second-hand smoke, such that in many cases some workers are still exposed to its toxic effects.

About half of the world's population (49%) is currently protected by national smoke-free policies that cover health-care and educational facilities, but only about 5% are protected by smoke-free laws that cover restaurants, pubs and bars.

About a third of countries protect their population from exposure to second-hand tobacco smoke with laws covering universities, and about 30% protect people at government facilities, but only 22% protect workers in indoor offices. About 30% of countries protect people with smoke-free legislation that covers public transport facilities; although smoking is frequently banned in transport vehicles, it is more likely to be permitted in stations as well as in semi-private vehicles such as taxis.

Few countries have good compliance with comprehensive smoke-free legislation

Good policy with inadequate compliance does not protect people from the dangers of second-hand tobacco smoke. Policy implementation must also be accompanied by a high level of compliance with those policies, so that the population is actually protected in fact and not merely theoretically protected on paper. Compliance with smoke-free policies varies greatly among countries, with comprehensive bans more likely to be complied with than smoke-free laws covering only some public places. Countries without comprehensive smoking bans are most likely to have the lowest levels of compliance.

Only 17 countries currently have smoke-free policies that provide universal and effective protection from second-hand smoke.

SMOKE-FREE ENVIRONMENTS – HIGHEST ACHIEVING COUNTRIES, 2008

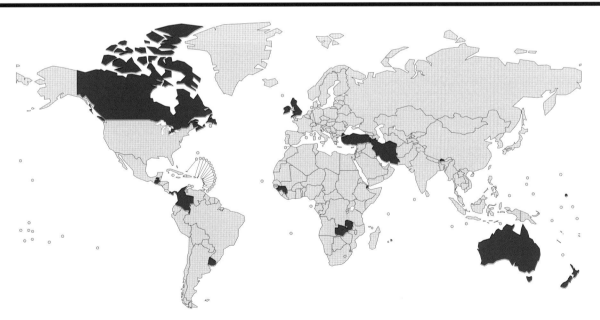

Wealthier countries are more likely to achieve high compliance with their comprehensive smoke-free legislation. Among high-income countries, four of five that have implemented comprehensive national smoke-free legislation have high compliance with the laws (with one country not reporting). Only three of 10 middle-income countries with comprehensive legislation have high compliance, and none of the two low-income countries with comprehensive laws have high compliance, suggesting that these laws are not fully protecting their citizens.

Compliance with smoke-free policies varies by type of location of the nearly half of countries that have policies in place (about 50%) report high levels of compliance in any one sector. Sectors with highest compliance reported are public transport (50% of countries have high compliance), indoor offices (49%), health-care facilities (42%), educational facilities except universities (38%), and restaurants (32%) and bars (30%).

Countries with comprehensive smoke-free laws are more likely to have strong enforcement provisions

For the first time in 2008, data were collected regarding existence of legal provisions for enforcement of smoke-free laws. Strong enforcement mechanisms for smoke-free laws – including provisions such as fining businesses or establishments who are in violation of the law and the presence of a complaints system to report violations – are most likely to have

been passed in higher-income countries. Of five high-income countries with comprehensive smoke-free laws, three have legislative language allowing clear, strong mechanisms for enforcement of their smoke-free law. In the middle-income group of countries, eight of ten with comprehensive smoking laws have strong enforcement mechanisms, as do one of two countries in the low-income group where all public places are smoke-free.

Smoke-free legislation at the subnational level

In 2008, data were collected for the first time regarding implementation of smoke-free legislation at the subnational level. Many countries have a government system in which state/provincial and local jurisdictions have significant legislative

Compliance with smoke-free policies varies greatly, with comprehensive bans more likely to be complied with than partial restrictions.

STATUS OF SMOKE-FREE LEGISLATION COVERING VARIOUS TYPES OF PUBLIC PLACES

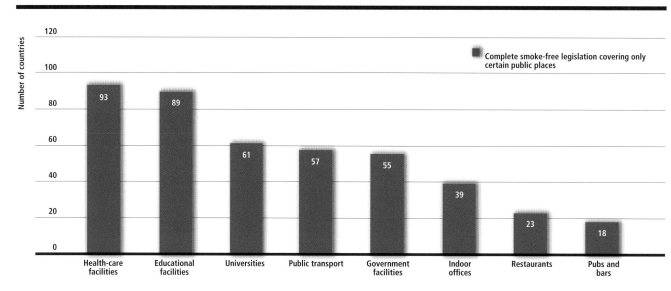

COUNTRY	POPULATION COVERED BY COMPLETE SMOKE-FREE LEGISLATION IN LARGE SUBNATIONAL JURISDICTIONS		TOTAL POPULATION (000)
	PERCENTAGE	NUMBER (000)	
United Kingdom of Great Britain and Northern Ireland	100	61 019	61 019
Canada	98	32 589	33 170
Australia	96	20 142	20 951
United Arab Emirates	29	1 292	4 503
United States of America	28	84 999	308 798
Central African Republic	14	623	4 424
Iraq	14	4 069	29 492
Argentina	12	4 813	39 934
Mexico	8	8 605	107 801
Switzerland	4	329	7 512
Venezuela (Bolivarian Republic of)	3	873	28 122
China	1	7 000	1 344 074
Total	3.4	226 320	World population: 6 741 434

power and have the ability to enact smoke-free legislation (and other laws) independently from national governments.

Among the large number of countries that have not enacted comprehensive smoke-free legislation at the national level, some subnational jurisdictions have been successful in enacting their own comprehensive smoke-free legislation. Often, it is more politically feasible to enact smoke-free legislation that covers a smaller population, such as a specific city or province. In some countries (notably Australia, Canada and the United States), governments at the state/provincial level have broad legislative powers, which in most other countries are reserved for the national government.

Currently, 7% of people in high-income countries are covered by comprehensive smoke-free legislation at the national level, and an additional 8% are covered at the subnational level. However, there has been almost no implementation of smoke-free legislation at the subnational level in middle- and low-income countries, despite many of these jurisdictions having the legal authority to do so.

If all subnational jurisdictions with the legal authority to implement comprehensive smoke-free policies were to do so, an additional 3.3 billion people would be protected from second-hand tobacco smoke. Among the population not currently protected by smoke-free legislation, 53% could potentially be protected through laws passed at the subnational level.

COMPLIANCE WITH SMOKE-FREE LEGISLATION BY LOCATION

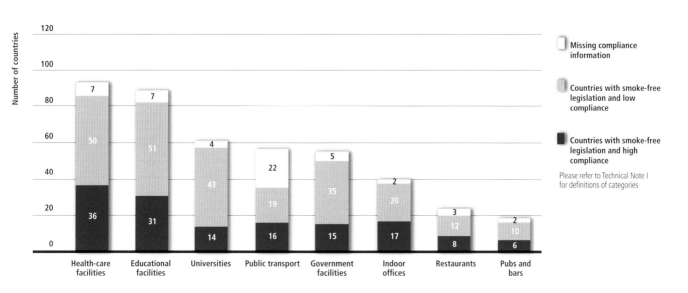

COMPLIANCE WITH COMPLETE SMOKE-FREE LEGISLATION

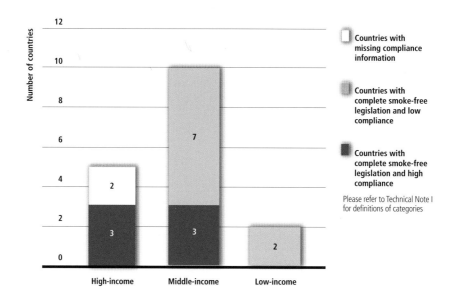

Countries with missing compliance information

Countries with complete smoke-free legislation and low compliance

Countries with complete smoke-free legislation and high compliance

Please refer to Technical Note I for definitions of categories

Smoke-free policy implementation must also be accompanied by a high level of compliance with those policies, so that the population is actually protected in fact and not merely theoretically protected on paper.

POTENTIAL FOR PROTECTING PEOPLE FROM SECOND-HAND TOBACCO SMOKE EXPOSURE AT THE SUBNATIONAL LEVEL

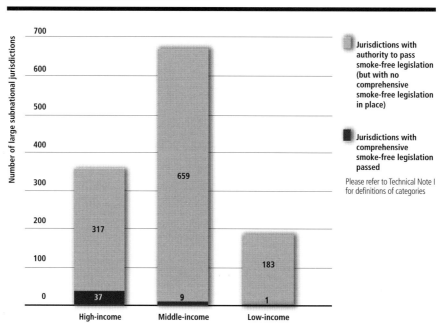

Jurisdictions with authority to pass smoke-free legislation (but with no comprehensive smoke-free legislation in place)

Jurisdictions with comprehensive smoke-free legislation passed

Please refer to Technical Note I for definitions of categories

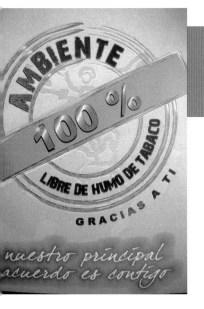

Mexico Federal District goes 100% smoke-free

Mexico Distrito Federal (Mexico City or Mexico DF), with a population of nearly 9 million, passed a comprehensive smoke-free law in February 2008. This law prohibits smoking in enclosed public places and workplaces, including public transport, restaurants and bars. Specifically, the law does not allow for designated smoking areas. Prior to passage of the law, nearly 40% of adult males and 17% of adult females reported current tobacco use, substantially higher than smoking rates in the rest of the country. Although limited smoke-free protections were in force prior to February 2008, they were nearly universally ignored.

Mexico DF's head of government and legislative assembly, along with support from tobacco control advocates, ensured that the 2008 smoke-free law protected all Mexico DF citizens from second-hand tobacco smoke. Working together, the Mexico DF government and tobacco control advocates secured strong support and active participation during all stages of the political process, enlisted civil society partners to coordinate actions in support of smoke-free laws, employed a high-profile media strategy that effectively engaged political and civil society advocates, and secured financial resources to implement promotional campaigns and research studies to support, inform and raise awareness of smoke-free agendas.

Public support for the law, which was extremely strong in the period leading up to enactment, solidified even further after smoke-free regulations came into force. More than 90% of Mexico DF residents now support restrictions in workplaces, restaurants and hotels, and more than 70% support the smoking ban in bars. The proportion of people reporting any exposure to second-hand tobacco smoke within the past month decreased from 80% to slightly over half, and daily exposure dropped from 28% to 12%. As smoke-free places have become firmly established, 98% of people polled agree that second-hand tobacco smoke is dangerous, 97% believe that the law benefits their health, and 98% concur that people have a right to breathe clean air.

By joining other large subnational jurisdictions that have become smoke-free, Mexico DF serves as a catalyst for similar action throughout Latin America and around the world.

Smoke-free laws in New Zealand are popular and well enforced

New Zealand, which has among the world's strongest tobacco control policies, first passed countrywide legislation in 1990 to restrict smoking in locations such as workplaces and schools. In December 2004, a comprehensive smoke-free law came into effect. It significantly strengthened the existing law, expanding it to cover all indoor workplaces, including hospitality venues (pubs, bars, restaurants and casinos), with no exemptions for designated smoking rooms.

Because an intensive educational campaign encouraged many of New Zealand's smokers to select the day the law went into effect as their quit date, there was a sharp upswing in demand for smoking cessation services in the period immediately afterwards. There were substantial increases in the number of calls to the national smokers' quit line and a 20% increase in the number of people receiving government subsidized nicotine replacement therapy.

The smoke-free law has been well accepted by the public, with support steadily strengthening since its introduction. In 2004, 61% of New Zealanders approved of the ban on smoking in bars, pubs and nightclubs, increasing to 74% in

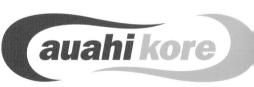

2005 and 82% in 2006. Support for the smoking ban in bars also increased significantly among smokers, from 29% in 2004 to 64% in 2006. Nearly 90% of people surveyed in 2006 supported the smoking ban in restaurants, as did 75% of smokers.

Studies have shown very high levels of compliance with the smoke-free law. The number of people reporting exposure to second-hand tobacco smoke in the workplace declined from 21% in 2004 to 8% in 2006, and bar patrons' exposure to second-hand tobacco smoke has dropped by about 90%. Legal action by health authorities for violations of the law has been rare, with fewer than 10 prosecutions. Contrary to warnings from opponents that the law would have serious economic effects on the hospitality industry, there has been no decrease in bar patronage or revenues.

Offer help to quit tobacco use

Treatment of tobacco dependence helps smokers quit and supports other tobacco control initiatives

It is difficult for the world's more than 1 billion tobacco users to quit. However, most smokers want to quit when informed of the health risks (127). Although most who quit eventually do so without intervention, assistance greatly increases quit rates (128). In November 2008, the Conference of the Parties asked a working group to develop guidelines to help Parties implement Article 14 of the WHO FCTC on cessation assistance and report to the Conference in 2010 (129).

Tobacco dependence treatment is primarily the responsibility of each country's health-care system (1). Despite their lower population-wide impact, individual cessation interventions have a significant impact on individual health and are extremely cost-effective compared with many other health system activities (130). People who quit smoking, regardless of their age, smoking history or health status, experience immediate and profound health benefits and can reduce most of the associated risks within a few years of quitting (131, 132).

Tobacco dependence treatment can include various methods, but programmes should include: cessation advice incorporated into primary health-care services; easily accessible and free telephone quit lines; and access to free or low-cost cessation medicines.

Integrated delivery of brief cessation counselling to tobacco users requires a well-functioning primary health-care system. Action to strengthen primary health care can draw on the WHO-developed health systems strengthening strategies to improve six health system building blocks (leadership/governance, health workforce, information support, medical products and technology, financing, and service delivery) (133). Brief cessation counselling is relatively inexpensive when integrated into existing primary health-care services, is usually well received by patients, and is most effective when it includes clear, strong and personalized advice to quit (128). There are many existing opportunities or entry points to incorporate brief cessation counselling into primary health-care services. Integration of brief cessation counselling into management and prevention of cardiovascular disease as well as tuberculosis care is already in process (134, 135). Doctors and other health-care workers should also serve as role models by not smoking themselves.

Advice and counselling can also be provided in the form of telephone quit lines, which should be free of charge and accessible to the public at convenient times (136).

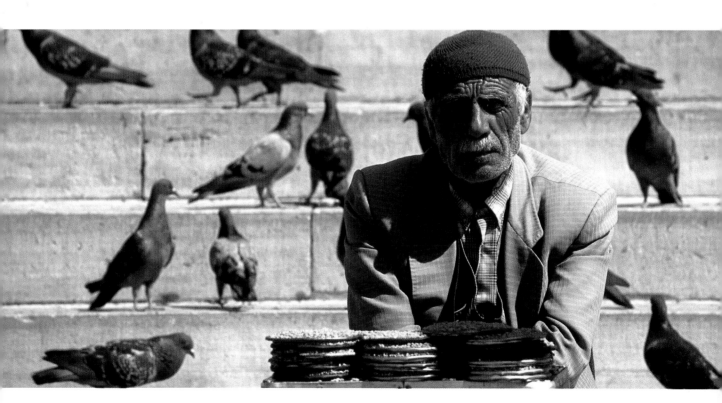

TOBACCO DEPENDENCE TREATMENT

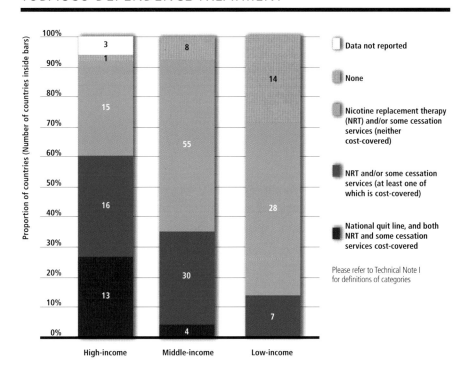

Proportion of countries (Number of countries inside bars)

High-income: 3, 1, 15, 16, 13
Middle-income: 8, 55, 30, 4
Low-income: 14, 28, 7

Legend:
- Data not reported
- None
- Nicotine replacement therapy (NRT) and/or some cessation services (neither cost-covered)
- NRT and/or some cessation services (at least one of which is cost-covered)
- National quit line, and both NRT and some cessation services cost-covered

Please refer to Technical Note I for definitions of categories

Smoking cessation services are most effective when they are part of a coordinated tobacco control programme.

TOBACCO DEPENDENCE TREATMENT – HIGHEST ACHIEVING COUNTRIES, 2008

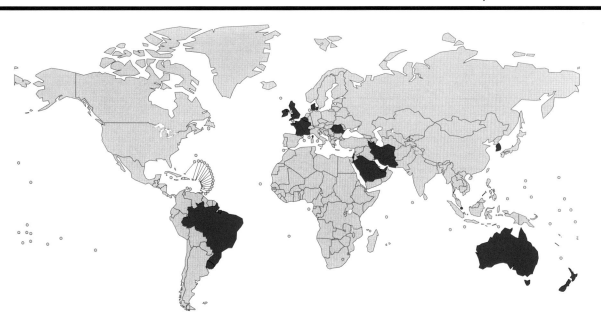

Pharmacological treatment of nicotine addiction should ideally be used in conjunction with advice and counselling, although it is also effective when provided separately (128). Cessation medications can double the likelihood that someone will successfully quit, and this probability increases even further if the medication is administered in conjunction with counselling. Nicotine replacement therapy (NRT) has recently been added to the 16th WHO Model List of Essential Medicines because of the high-quality evidence of its effectiveness, acceptable safety and cost-effectiveness (137). At least some forms of NRT should be broadly available at very affordable prices to the tobacco user wanting to quit.

Smoking cessation services are most effective when they are part of a coordinated tobacco control programme. Wealthy countries with substantial financial resources should be expected to offer comprehensive quit smoking services at no or minimal cost, although low- and medium-income countries can effectively implement at least some cessation services. Most countries can use lower-cost counselling options effectively, even when financial support for medications is beyond

budgetary limits. Uruguay, an example of a middle-income country that has a strong commitment to effective tobacco control, has implemented some components of a comprehensive cessation programme. Although Uruguay covers the cost of some types of NRT and other medications, it does not cover other types due to cost constraints. While Uruguay has developed national treatment guidelines and provides extensive counselling services, there is currently no national quit line or formal mechanism for provision of physician counselling in primary care, although these services are planned for the near future when funding is made available. Governments can use tobacco tax revenues to fund quit lines and subsidize clinical cessation services, and providing cessation support may also reduce opposition to other tobacco control policies.

Only 17 countries provide access to comprehensive help to quit smoking

- Three countries (Israel, Romania and United Arab Emirates) joined the group of countries offering comprehensive help to quit smoking in 2008, bringing

the total number with a national quit line and coverage for costs of both NRT and some cessation services to 17, covering 8.2% of the world's population (compared with 7.7% in 2007).

- High-income countries have made the greatest progress in offering help for people who want to quit tobacco use, with 27% operating a national quit line and at least partially covering the cost of the cost of both NRT and some cessation services. High-income countries are most able to afford to cover these costs.

- About a third of middle-income countries and less than 15% of low-income countries provide coverage for NRT and/ or cessation services. Only four middle-income countries and no low-income countries provide a national toll-free quit line and coverage for both NRT and cessation services.

- In the vast majority of low- and middle-income countries, the cost of cessation assistance is not covered by government, and 8% of middle-income and 29% of low-income countries provide no assistance to smokers at all.

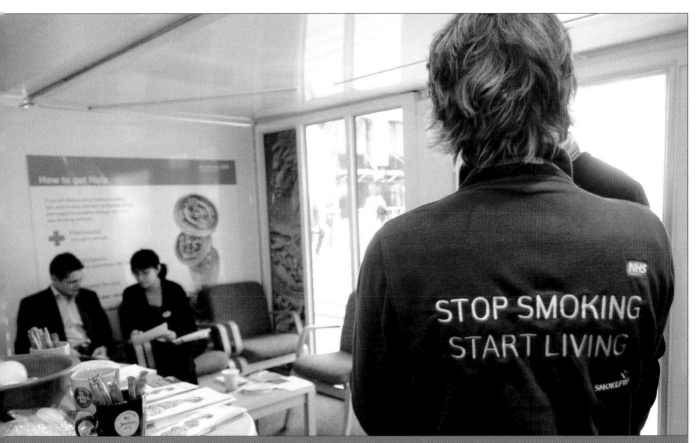

England provides free, comprehensive tobacco dependence treatment to all

The four countries of the United Kingdom of Great Britain and Northern Ireland have a national tobacco dependence treatment service that is universally available to all smokers, mainly free of charge, through the countries' National Health Service (NHS).

In England for example, nicotine replacement therapy (NRT) is available without prescription through pharmacies and in other stores (e.g. supermarkets and corner shops). NRT, as well as other smoking cessation medications, is also available by prescription at a reduced charge. Because people with low incomes are exempt from prescription charges, all prescription medicines including NRT, Bupropion and Varenicline are free to around half of England's population, with the remainder paying a small charge equivalent to about US$ 10 for about one month of medications (although this can vary).

There are also two free national quit lines – one operated through the NHS and a separate one run by an independent organization called Quit. The NHS Stop Smoking Helpline is available 16 hours a day, 7 days a week. Callers are offered counselling on the telephone, are proactively called back or sent e-mails or text messages to provide ongoing support and motivation, and are given details about their local treatment services. The NHS Asian Tobacco Helpline,

available one day a week, provides similar services in five languages (Bengali, Gujarati, Hindi, Punjabi and Urdu).

Any smoker can go to his or her general practitioner and be referred to specialized treatment or go directly to a treatment centre, at no charge. To further improve treatment services, England has launched a national training centre that will develop evidence-based training for stop smoking counsellors and managers, assess core competences and certify counsellors, and commission and accredit training. An evaluation found that treatment services disproportionately reach low-income smokers in England – the opposite of what usually happens with health promotion – which means that these services are helping those most in need. For additional information on tobacco dependence treatment in England please refer to http://smokefree.nhs.uk/.

This is an example of what is possible with a significant investment of resources. For low- and middle-income countries that do not have the financial resources to support implementation of a comprehensive cessation programme, there are steps that can be taken to help people quit while more comprehensive initiatives are developed as mentioned above in the case of Uruguay.

Warn about the dangers of tobacco

Warning labels on tobacco packaging and hard-hitting mass media campaigns provide needed information about the health dangers of smoking

Despite conclusive evidence regarding the dangers of tobacco, relatively few tobacco users worldwide understand the full extent of the risk to their health (*138*). Smokers tend to underestimate the risks of tobacco use to themselves and others. Article 11 (*Packaging and labelling of tobacco products*) of the WHO FCTC establishes an obligation for Parties to meet global standards for warning labels that clearly communicate the dangers of tobacco use in the principal national language, comprise not less than 30% of the principal display areas on all tobacco products, and rotate periodically. The Conference of the Parties has developed and adopted guidelines for implementing Article 11 (*3*).

Comprehensive warnings about the dangers of tobacco are critical to changing tobacco's image, especially among adolescents and young adults, the ages at which people are most likely to begin tobacco use (*139*). Ultimately, the objective of anti-tobacco education and counter-advertising is to change social norms about tobacco use. This will cause many individuals to choose not to use tobacco, and also increases support for other tobacco control measures. Article 12 (*Education, communication, training and public awareness*) of the WHO FCTC reinforces this by creating a legal obligation for Parties to promote access to information about the dangers of tobacco consumption and the benefits of cessation. To this end, a working group is elaborating guidelines for implementation of Article 12 for adoption by the Conference of the Parties (*140*).

Prominent warning labels on tobacco product packaging provide the most direct health messages to all smokers, as well as to non-smokers who see the packs (*138, 141-143*). Warning labels encourage smokers to quit and discourage non-smokers from starting, are well accepted by the public, and can be implemented at virtually no cost to governments. Warnings on both the front and back of packaging are extremely important so that smokers cannot overlook them, but most countries do not require warning labels of this size on both sides of packaging.

Warning labels should describe specific health effects and diseases caused by tobacco use, and should be periodically rotated to continue to attract the attention of the public. Pictorial warnings are more effective than text-only warnings (*143*), and are essential for persons who cannot read and for young children whose parents smoke. Deceptive terms such as "low tar", "light", or "mild" should also be banned; these terms suggest incorrectly that some products are less harmful (*144*).

HEALTH WARNINGS

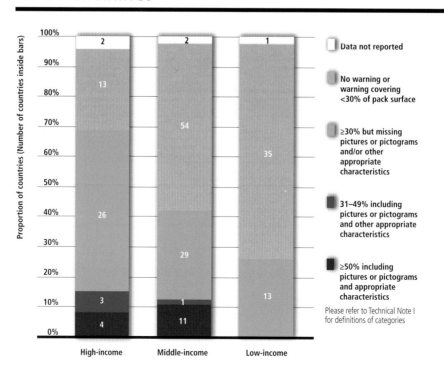

Anti-tobacco advertising in all forms of media can help publicize the full extent of tobacco's dangers and can counter tobacco use as a social norm. When exposed to effective television anti-tobacco messages, teenagers are half as likely to become established smokers (*145*) and adult smokers are more likely to quit (*146*). Hard-hitting campaigns using graphic images that demonstrate the physical harm caused by tobacco use are especially effective in convincing users to quit (*147*). The tobacco industry has created its own anti-tobacco advertising, but its advertisements are ineffective in reducing smoking and may even increase smoking, especially among the young (*148*). In addition to paid advertising, anti-tobacco educational campaigns can also be supplemented effectively and inexpensively through public relations efforts that generate free media coverage (a process sometimes referred to as "earned media") (*149*).

Only 8% of the world's population live in a country with strong graphic warnings on cigarette packs

- Five countries (Djibouti, Egypt, Iran, Malaysia and Mauritius, totalling 178 million people) joined the group of countries that fully meet WHO FCTC Article 11 guidelines for pack warning labels in 2008. Fifteen countries covering 7.6% of the world's population (compared with 4.9% in 2007) now require warning labels that cover at least half of both the front and back of cigarette packs and also include pictures and all other listed characteristics.
- All of the countries newly implementing comprehensive warning label requirements in 2008 were middle-income countries.
- Less than 10% of high-income countries require warning labels with all appropriate characteristics. Although more than a quarter of low-income countries have warning labels covering at least 30% of packages, all are missing other important characteristics – most notably, they lack pictures or pictograms that can be easily understood by people who are less educated or who are unable to read.
- More than 70% of low-income countries and nearly 55% of middle-income countries require either no warning labels of any kind or labels that cover less than 30% of cigarette packs.
- In most countries, there are essentially no health warnings at all on smoked tobacco products other than manufactured cigarettes (e.g. bidis, kreteks, roll-your-own and water pipe tobacco). Only one high-income country and six middle-income countries require strong health warnings on these other smoked tobacco products.

WARN ABOUT THE DANGERS OF TOBACCO – HIGHEST ACHIEVING COUNTRIES, 2008

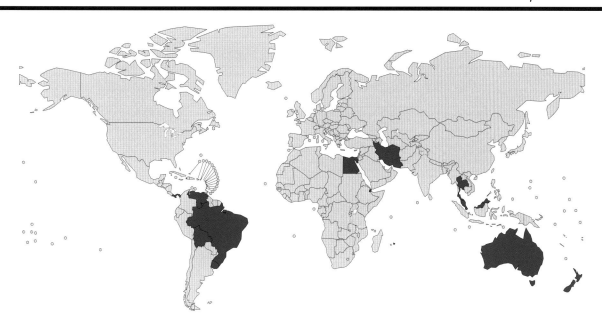

Five countries totalling 178 million people adopted graphic health warnings on cigarette packs in 2008.

Mass media campaign in India

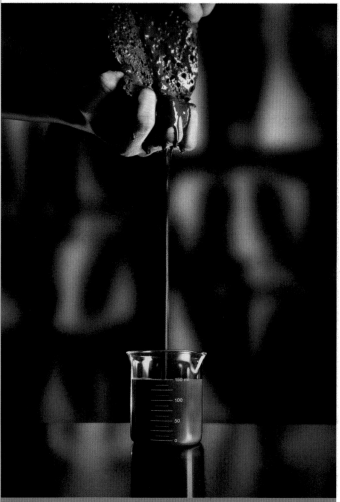

Image from "Sponge" TV campaign in India. "Lungs are like sponges. Smokers' lungs are like sponges full of tar."

As part of a systematic strengthening of its national tobacco control programme, India has implemented several mass media advertising campaigns. These intend to increase public awareness of the harms of smoking and second-hand tobacco smoke, change attitudes towards tobacco use, and motivate smokers to quit. As with pack warning labels, public service announcements should be rotated periodically so that they maintain their impact.

In its most recent campaign, India ran the advertisement "Sponge", which was originally developed by the Cancer Institute New South Wales (Australia). It graphically depicts the amount of cancer-producing tar that an average smoker's lungs soak up in just one year. This vivid demonstration illustrates that smoking is more harmful than many people realize.

The Sponge campaign was adapted and aired in five languages: the original English, with translations into Bengali, Gujarati, Hindi and Tamil. The Government of India spent approximately US$ 1 million to purchase television advertising time for Sponge spots, which ran on 40 national and regional television channels for a six-week period in June and July 2009.

The campaign was rigorously tested among 24 local focus groups to ensure it resonated similarly with Indian audiences. Among the 10 tobacco control advertisements tested, Sponge ranked highest in terms of behavioural indicators, such as making smokers concerned about their smoking, more likely to quit, and more likely to speak to someone about stopping smoking.

These pre-testing efforts are critical to the success of mass media campaigns, because cultural differences and belief systems can play a role in how messages are received, and must be considered before publicity can be promoted in a particular country.

In India, where 10% of the world's smokers live, nearly a million people are killed by tobacco-related diseases each year. About a third of Indian men smoke cigarettes or bidis, and more than half either smoke or use chewing tobacco. Tobacco use among women, while historically low, is increasing, as are smoking rates among youth.

Earned media efforts target tobacco promotion and sponsorship in Indonesia

In Indonesia, the tobacco industry is poorly regulated. Legislation banning tobacco advertising and marketing is weak, as are laws that establish smoke-free places and require health warnings on cigarette packaging, and tobacco industry interests are well represented in government. As a result, major multinational tobacco companies are free to employ marketing tactics that they are prohibited from using elsewhere.

Tobacco company sponsorship of events that target youth and young adults can be especially difficult to monitor and regulate, even in countries that have enacted strong tobacco control legislation. Several Indonesian nongovernmental organizations have successfully developed and implemented strategies focused on earned media, which involves outreach to journalists to generate news stories in print and broadcast media.

In July 2008, Indonesian nongovernmental organizations contacted popular singer Alicia Keys to ask her to withdraw tobacco industry sponsorship of her concert in Jakarta and to speak out against the tobacco industry. The story was pitched to international media outlets, generating a number of news stories in both international and Indonesian media. As a result of this coverage, Keys immediately demanded that the tobacco sponsorship be withdrawn, and the sponsoring company (Philip Morris International) agreed to remove billboards and posters promoting its involvement.

Other successes resulting from earned media range from stopping promotional activities and giveaways of free cigarette samples at concerts, forcing withdrawal of tobacco companies from sponsorship of high-profile music festivals, and highlighting marketing of tobacco products directly to children.

Komoditas Penuh Tipu Daya

Iran implements strong pack warning labels

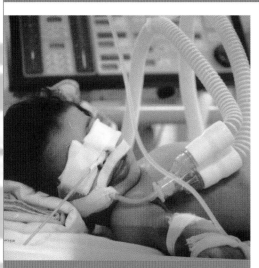

Iran cigarette package warning

To combat the continuing problem of tobacco use, the Islamic Republic of Iran enacted a comprehensive national tobacco control law in 2006 that established a national tobacco control programme headed by the ministry of health, banned all types of direct and indirect tobacco advertising and marketing, implemented an ongoing series of annual tax increases, and mandated strong health warnings on cigarette packaging, among other interventions.

In 2008, the Islamic Republic of Iran further strengthened its law to require pictorial warnings on all cigarette packages sold in the country beginning in January 2009. These warning labels cover 50% of both the front and back of all cigarette packages and incorporate graphic, full-colour images of diseases caused by smoking. Eight health warnings have been approved for use and will be rotated on cigarette packages over a period of two years, when another set of graphic warning labels will be introduced. Use of misleading terms, such as "mild" and "light", are also banned. As a result, Iran's requirements now fully meet the WHO FCTC Article 11 guidelines for size, content and presentation of cigarette pack warning labels, and thus effectively warn smokers about the risks to their health.

mpower Enforce bans on tobacco advertising, promotion and sponsorship

Banning tobacco advertising, promotion and sponsorship reduces smoking and denormalizes tobacco use

The tobacco industry spends tens of billions of dollars worldwide each year on advertising, promotion and sponsorship (*150*). To counter this, WHO FCTC Article 13 (*Tobacco advertising, promotion and sponsorship*) calls for comprehensive bans on tobacco advertising, promotion and sponsorship in accordance with each country's constitutional principles (*1*). To assist countries in achieving this goal, the Conference of the Parties adopted guidelines for implementing Article 13 (*3*).

Tobacco advertising, promotion and sponsorship can make smoking more socially acceptable, impede efforts to educate people about the hazards

of tobacco use, and strengthen the tobacco industry's influence over media, sporting and entertainment businesses. A comprehensive ban on all advertising, promotion and sponsorship protects people from industry marketing tactics and could decrease tobacco consumption by about 7%, independent of other tobacco control interventions (*151*). Complete bans block the industry's ability to continue marketing to young people who have not yet started to use tobacco, and to adult tobacco users who want to quit. Partial bans have little or no effect: if advertising is prohibited in a particular medium, the tobacco industry merely redirects expenditures to places where advertising is permitted (*152, 153*).

The tobacco industry strongly opposes marketing bans because they are highly effective in reducing tobacco use. The industry often argues that outright bans

on advertising, promotion and sponsorship are not necessary and that voluntary codes and self-regulation are sufficient. However, voluntary restrictions are ineffective because there is no force of law, and ultimately the industry fails to comply with its own voluntary regulations (*154*). Government intervention through well-drafted and well-enforced legislation is required because the tobacco industry has substantial expertise in circumventing advertising bans.

Only Panama implemented a new ban on tobacco advertising, promotion and sponsorship in 2008

- One country (Panama) joined the group of countries with complete bans on all forms of advertising, promotion and

BANS ON ADVERTISING, PROMOTION AND SPONSORSHIP

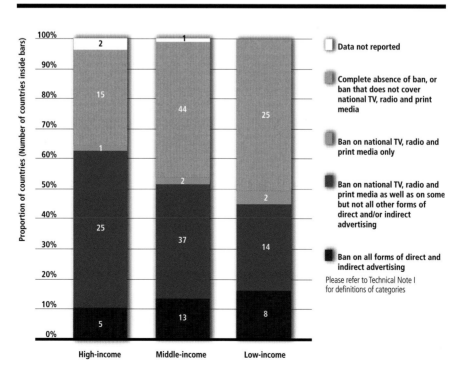

COVERAGE AND COMPLIANCE WITH COMPREHENSIVE BANS ON TOBACCO ADVERTISING, PROMOTION AND SPONSORSHIP

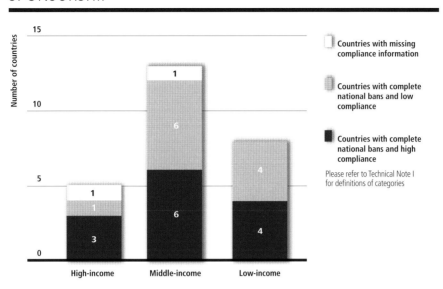

Legend:
- Countries with missing compliance information
- Countries with complete national bans and low compliance
- Countries with complete national bans and high compliance

Please refer to Technical Note I for definitions of categories

A comprehensive ban on all advertising, promotion and sponsorship protects people from industry marketing tactics and could decrease tobacco consumption by about 7%.

ENFORCE BANS ON TOBACCO ADVERTISING, PROMOTION AND SPONSORSHIP – HIGHEST ACHIEVING COUNTRIES, 2008

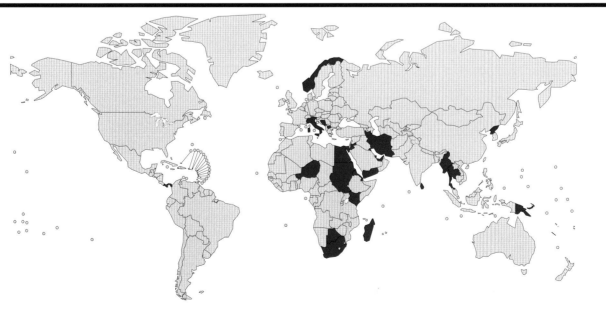

sponsorship in 2008, bringing the total number with complete bans on all forms of direct and indirect advertising and marketing to 26, covering 8.8% of the world's population (compared with 8.7% in 2007).

- Middle-income countries have made greater progress in implementing comprehensive bans on all advertising, promotion and sponsorship than have low- or high-income countries.

- More than half of high-income countries have banned tobacco advertising in all broadcast and print media but ban only some other forms of direct and indirect advertising, compared with over one third of middle-income countries and about 28% of low-income countries.

- Few countries with comprehensive bans on tobacco advertising, promotion and sponsorship enforce these policies to a high degree. Only three high-income countries and six middle-income countries have achieved high compliance, and four low-income country have done so.

Low- and middle-income countries are more likely than high-income countries to have comprehensive bans on all tobacco advertising, promotion and sponsorship.

Jordan strengthens prohibitions on tobacco advertising, promotion and sponsorship

Jordan, which first began to implement tobacco control measures more than 30 years ago, further strengthened its restrictions on tobacco advertising, promotion and sponsorship in 2008. All tobacco advertising and marketing activities had in theory been banned starting in 1977, but enforcement of these and other tobacco control provisions was generally weak. Although the ban on marketing and promotion of tobacco products was adequately enforced, the judiciary tended not to prosecute violations vigorously and frequently imposed only the minimum permissible penalties, thus leading to widespread violations.

The 2008 legislation clarified and strengthened the wording of Jordan's tobacco control laws, dedicated additional resources to tobacco control, and increased training of tobacco control programme staff. Additionally, the law added several new provisions to limit point-of-sale tobacco marketing, including bans on the sale of individual cigarettes and sales through vending machines.

To strengthen enforcement, the ministry of health trained 35 health promotion coordinators regarding the tobacco control legislation, practical and suitable methods for enforcing and implementing the law, and procedures for inspections. These coordinators have broad authority to warn and educate people about the law, confiscate any prohibited promotional materials, and initiate judicial proceedings to enforce the laws.

The capital city of Amman, where the full range of tobacco promotional activities used to be pervasive, was selected to pilot these new provisions. In Amman today, print and electronic media are now free from tobacco advertising, tobacco billboards are gone, there is no tobacco sponsorship of sports or cultural activities, and tobacco vending machines have disappeared. This successful model for enforcing advertising and marketing bans is now ready to be expanded to the rest of the country.

Panama bans all tobacco advertising, promotion and sponsorship

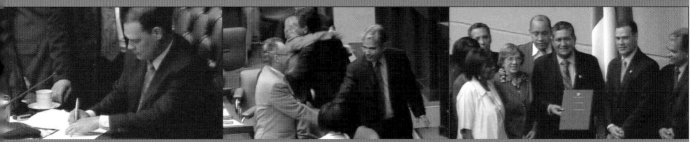

Signing of the legislation

In 2008, Panama became the first country in the Americas to enact a total ban on all advertising, promotion and sponsorship of tobacco products. Before implementing its new law, Panama had virtually no restrictions of any kind on tobacco advertising and marketing. The new law completely bans all forms of direct or indirect tobacco advertising and marketing, including distribution of clothing and other items with tobacco brand logos as well as sponsorship of sports teams and other high-profile events that often involve children. Advertising in international media originating outside the country is also prohibited.

In addition to banning advertising in all media, including outdoor displays such as billboards, Panama's law also prohibits distribution of free tobacco products, promotional price discounting, and product placement in television and motion pictures. Of particular note is the restriction on advertising and marketing at the point of sale, which

most countries with even comprehensive bans have been unable to pass. The tobacco industry has already found loopholes in the law banning point-of-sale marketing, which highlights the tobacco industry's willingness to violate the spirit of the law to market its products, as well as the need for tobacco control experts to closely monitor industry activities.

The most comprehensive ban on advertising and marketing will have little effect if it is not enforced. Even though Panama's law has been in place for less than two years, levels of compliance are extremely high, ranking 95 out of a possible 100 points. In a recent assessment of compliance with the law, several neighbourhoods of Panama City as well as rural areas of the country were surveyed. In all areas visited, no advertising of any kind was seen, no indirect promotion or sponsorship activities were observed, and only one violation of the point-of-sale marketing ban was noted.

Madagascar passes legislation banning all tobacco advertising, promotion and sponsorship

Madagascar has had moderately strong tobacco control policies in place for the last few years. In addition to a ban on smoking in public places and health warnings that cover 50% of tobacco packaging, all tobacco advertising, promotion and sponsorship activities are prohibited. Both direct advertising and indirect marketing are covered by the ban.

Because the law prohibiting tobacco advertising, promotion and sponsorship has been well enforced and includes strict penalties

for violations, these activities have ceased completely. Throughout Madagascar, there are no television, newspaper, magazine or billboard advertisements for tobacco products, and Internet marketing is similarly banned. Promotional activities such as distribution of free cigarettes and tobacco product rewards have ended. To strengthen monitoring and enforcement, district-level public health officials and local law enforcement work closely with the national tobacco control programme and the ministry of health to expose and investigate violations.

Raise taxes on tobacco

Increasing the price of tobacco is the most effective intervention to reduce smoking

Increasing the price of tobacco products through significant tax increases is the single most effective way to decrease tobacco use and to encourage current users to quit (*155*). In addition, higher tobacco taxes are particularly effective in keeping youth from taking up tobacco use and in reducing use among the poor (*156*), as both groups are highly responsive to price changes (*155-157*). In Article 6 (*Price and tax measures to reduce the demand for tobacco*) the WHO FCTC recognizes the effectiveness of raising taxes on tobacco products.

Governments levy many taxes on tobacco products, including excise taxes, value added and other sales taxes, and import duties. Among these, excises are the most important due to their specificity to tobacco products. There are two types of excise taxes: specific excises (based on quantity, weight and/or other characteristics) and ad valorem excises (based on value). High specific excises are the most appropriate method to protect public health, since these lead to relatively higher prices and smaller price differences between premium and discount brands, which will result in reduced tobacco use.

Cigarettes should become less affordable over time to reduce consumption

To improve public health, tobacco taxes should also make tobacco products progressively less affordable by offsetting the combined effects of inflation and increased consumer incomes and purchasing power. This requires periodic increases in specific excise taxes to maintain their impact. Many countries have tobacco products that are becoming increasingly more affordable because taxes do not keep pace with inflation and incomes.

As demonstrated in country after country, increasing tobacco taxes increases tobacco tax revenues in the short and medium term, even when taking reduced consumption into account (*155*). This is due to relatively low price sensitivity of demand; in high-income countries, a 10% increase in tobacco prices reduces consumption by about 4% (*158*), with larger reductions expected in lower-income countries where price sensitivity is likely to be greater. Price increases are particularly effective where there is a low share of taxes contributing to retail prices.

For the greatest revenue impact, the overall tax structure should be simple and easy to implement. A more complex structure is likely to increase tax evasion and tax avoidance. For specific excises, the risk of tax avoidance is increased when the tax is based on product characteristics (e.g. length or weight) rather than quantity. Ad valorem excises maintain their value adjusted to inflation, while specific excises need to be regularly adjusted to keep pace with inflation; to date, only two countries (Australia and New Zealand) automatically adjust their specific excises for inflation.

Contrary to tobacco industry's claims, increased smuggling does not

TOTAL TAX ON CIGARETTES

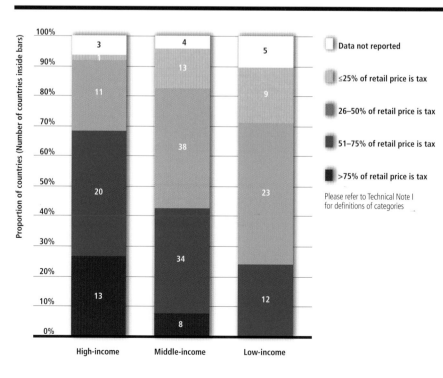

automatically follow tax increases (*159*). Large tobacco tax and price increases in several countries have not been followed by dramatic increases in smuggling. Other factors, such as weak border controls, poor tax administration, the presence of informal distribution channels, and people's willingness to buy smuggled products can be more important determinants of smuggling than differences in tax rates. Many countries with high taxes and prices (e.g. Finland, Norway and Sweden) show relatively little evidence of smuggling, while several low tax and price countries (e.g. Italy and Spain) experience a relatively higher incidence of smuggling (*159*).

Tax compliance is facilitated by a centralized system that focuses on manufacturers with strong tax administration and customs enforcement. Article 15 (*Illicit trade in tobacco products*) of the WHO FCTC states that monitoring tobacco production and trade can contribute to reducing illicit trade; furthermore, the currently negotiated draft protocol on illicit trade in tobacco products proposes to control and monitor tobacco production and trade to eliminate illicit trade (*160*).

In 2008, there was a minimal increase in the proportion of the world's population covered by effective tobacco taxation policies

- Six more countries (Czech Republic, Estonia, Fiji, Finland, the Netherlands, and Seychelles) joined the group of countries that levy taxes higher than 75% of retail price in 2008, bringing the total number that levy taxes at this rate to 21, covering 6.2% of the world's population (compared with 5.7% in 2007).
- Globally, the average total tax contribution to total retail prices of tobacco products was just under 50% in 2008.
- Tax rates are generally highest in high-income countries. The average contribution of total taxes to the total retail price of cigarettes is 63% in high-income countries, 49% in middle-income countries, and 39% in low-income countries.
- About 70% of high-income countries levy taxes that account for at least half of the total tax-inclusive retail sales price, compared with less than half of middle-income countries and about 25% of low-income countries. Relatively few countries (13 high-income, eight middle-income, and no low-income) impose excise and other taxes on cigarettes that account for at least 75% of retail price.
- Cigarettes are more than twice as expensive in high-income countries as in middle-income countries, and nearly five times as expensive as in low-income countries.
- Of 163 countries for which cigarette excise tax data are available, 55 countries rely solely on specific excises and 60 countries solely on ad valorem excises, 48 countries (mostly in Europe) use a combination of the two, and 19 countries impose no excise tax but instead rely on import duties on cigarettes instead.

RAISE TAXES ON TOBACCO – HIGHEST ACHIEVING COUNTRIES, 2008

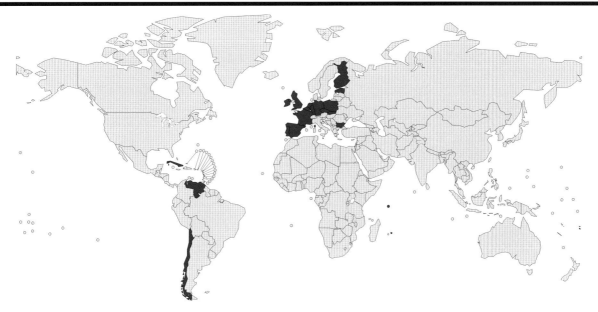

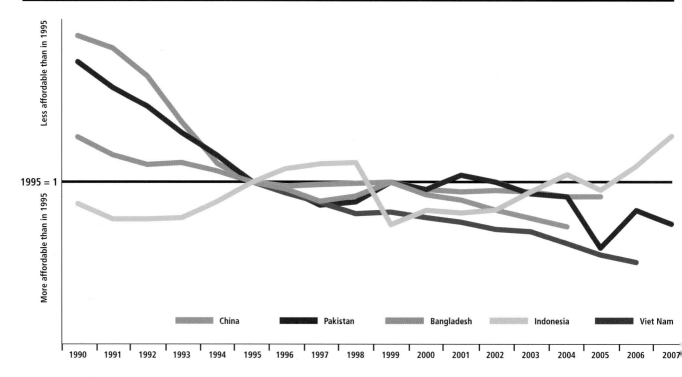

Source: WHO calculations using data from papers prepared as part of the Bloomberg Initiative to Reduce Tobacco Use (published at http://www.worldlungfoundation.org/publications.ph)

Note: The affordability index is created by first dividing the price of the most popular brand by the average per capita income (GDP/capita). The value for 1995 is assumed to be 1 and the values of other years are estimated by using 1995 as a base. The estimated values greater than 1 indicate that cigarettes were less affordable compared with the 1995 level. Similarly, the estimated values that are less than 1 indicate that cigarettes were more affordable compared with the 1995 level.

Increasing the price of tobacco products through significant tax increases is the single most effective way to decrease tobacco use and to encourage current users to quit.

AVERAGE RETAIL PRICE AND TAXATION (EXCISE AND TOTAL) OF MOST SOLD BRANDS OF CIGARETTES, 2008

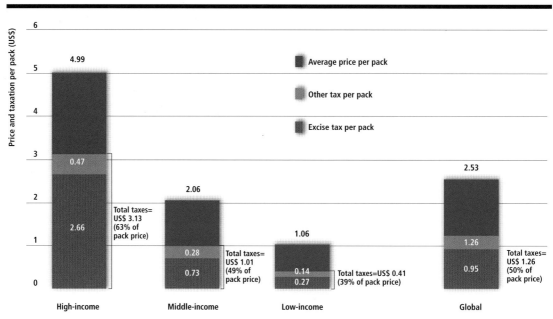

Thailand earmarks tobacco tax revenues for tobacco control

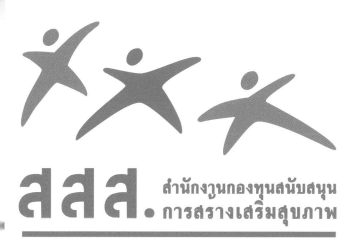

Thailand, a leader in tobacco control, levied an 83.5% statutory excise tax on cigarettes, which in 2008 resulted in an overall tax rate of 57% of the actual retail pack price. An important feature of Thailand's tax structure is a 2% tax surcharge, collected on both tobacco and alcohol, that is earmarked for a broad agenda of national health promotion programs. The 2% excise earmark, established in Thailand's Health Promotion Foundation Act of 2001, secures funding for the Thai Health Promotion Foundation (ThaiHealth) and provides annual revenues of about US$ 35 million.

With this funding, ThaiHealth seeks to reduce sickness and death and make general improvements in quality of life.

Another strong feature of Thailand's cigarette tax structure is that cigarette excise taxes have been increased more rapidly than the inflation rate. As a result, the relative affordability of cigarettes has decreased. In January 1992, at a time when adult smoking prevalence was 30% (nearly 60% among males), the excise rate was set at 55%. The tax rate was increased to the current 83.5% in a series of eight steps, which increased the retail price of the most popular brand by nearly 400% and nearly tripled Thailand's annual tobacco tax revenues. Adult smoking rates have now decreased to about 18%, with youth male smoking rates about half of adult male rates.

Thailand levies taxes on all cigarette products at a single rate, which simplifies calculation and collection of taxes. Because the domestic tobacco industry is state-controlled, the government can set the wholesale factory price, thus ensuring that manufacturers are unable to reduce prices to counter the effects of increased taxation. Industry price manipulation is an important concern in countries that rely solely on ad valorem tax and that do not have a state-controlled tobacco industry.

EXCISE TAX RATE, EXCISE REVENUE AND SMOKING PREVALENCE, THAILAND, 1991–2007

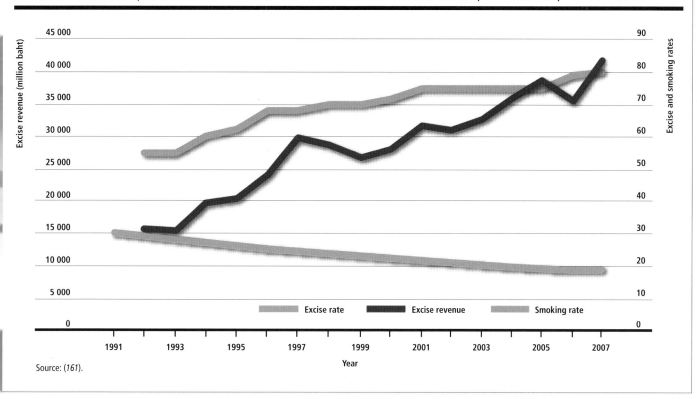

Source: (161).

National tobacco control programmes and capacity

National programmes are required to lead tobacco control efforts

Building national capacity to carry out effective and sustainable national tobacco control programmes is critical to reversing the tobacco epidemic, and countries are obligated to implement a national tobacco control programme as part of their WHO FCTC obligations (1). Nongovernmental organizations and other members of civil society not affiliated with the tobacco industry, including health professional bodies, women's, youth, environmental and consumer groups, and academic and health-care institutions, have made great contributions to tobacco control efforts nationally and internationally. Although involvement by many sectors of government and civil society is required to implement an effective national tobacco control programme, strategic planning and leadership should occur centrally within a country's ministry of health (57). In larger countries, the programme may be designed for flexible implementation by decentralizing authority to subnational jurisdictions (57).

A national tobacco control programme with full-time, dedicated staff at both central and (where appropriate) subnational levels, with support from senior levels throughout government as well as technical experts and persons with expertise in planning and implementation, can provide highly effective leadership and administration of all programme initiatives. Additionally, a national coordinating committee for tobacco control convened at a high level of government (i.e. cabinet or presidency) should include representatives from all government and civil society groups directly involved with tobacco control activities.

It is critical that the government provide its tobacco control programme with a steady source of funding at both national and, where appropriate, subnational levels. Because most governments currently collect hundreds or even thousands of times more in tobacco tax revenues than they spend on tobacco control, there is room to increase tobacco control spending substantially. This can be accomplished either through use of general government funds or specific earmarks from tobacco tax revenues. Other sources of funding include donations and grants from national and international nongovernmental or philanthropic organizations.

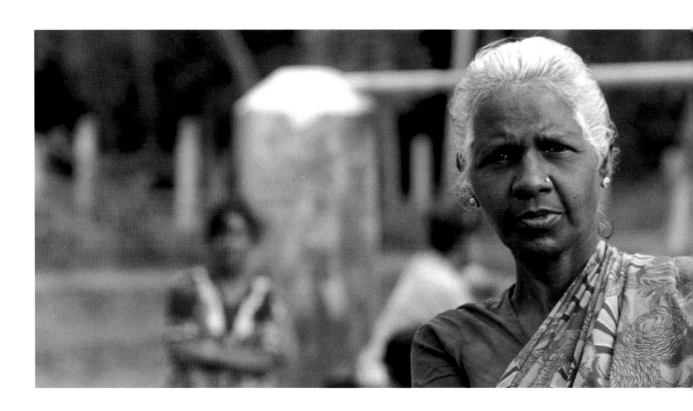

TOBACCO CONTROL IS UNDERFUNDED

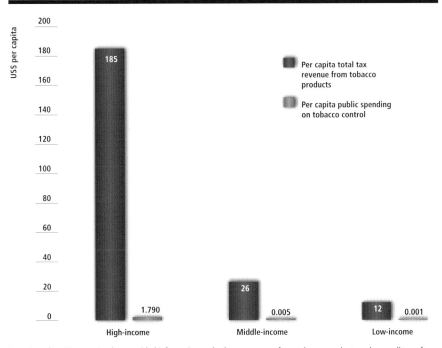

US$ per capita

- 185 — High-income
- 1.790 — High-income
- 26 — Middle-income
- 0.005 — Middle-income
- 12 — Low-income
- 0.001 — Low-income

■ Per capita total tax revenue from tobacco products

▨ Per capita public spending on tobacco control

Note: Based on 55 countries that provided information on both tax revenues from tobacco products and expenditures for tobacco control for 2007 and 2008.

Governments annually collect more than US$ 167 billion in tobacco tax revenues, yet spend a total of only US$ 965 million on tobacco control.

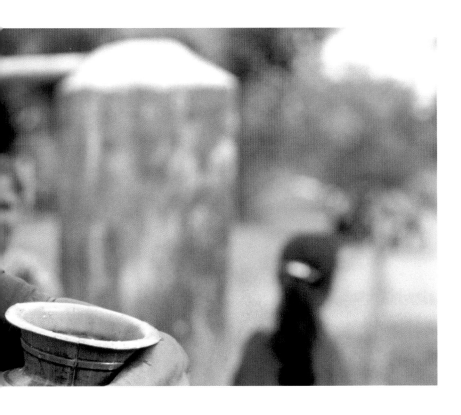

Data from 2007 and 2008 show that aggregate tobacco tax revenues in countries reporting data are more than 173 times higher than expenses for tobacco control activities. Governments collect annually more than US$ 167 billion in tobacco tax revenues, yet spend a total of only US$ 965 million on tobacco control – with 99% of this amount spent by 17 high-income countries. Per capita spending on tobacco control ranges from a tenth of a cent per capita per year in low-income countries to half a cent per capita per year in middle-income countries and about US$ 1.80 per capita per year in high-income countries.

Most countries have a national tobacco control programme, but many do not staff them adequately

- Nearly 80% of countries report having a national agency with responsibility for tobacco control objectives, with low- and middle-income countries more likely to have such an agency than high-income countries.
- Less than 15% of high-income countries and 22% of middle-income countries also have an agency with at least five full-time equivalent staff members, while 24% of low-income countries have an agency staffed at that level.

NATIONAL TOBACCO CONTROL PROGRAMMES

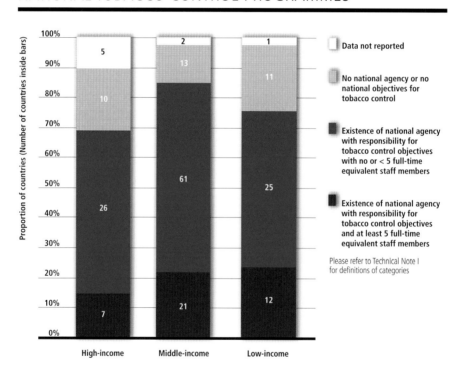

It is critical that governments provide tobacco control programmes with a steady source of funding at both national and, where appropriate, subnational levels.

Brazil has high capacity in tobacco control programmes

Brazil has given high priority and commitment to combating the tobacco epidemic. The country's comprehensive approach to tobacco control is based on a sector-wide national coordination mechanism, which is led by a national tobacco control programme under the ministry of health that serves as the secretariat of the tobacco control health sector commission and the national committee for implementation of the WHO FCTC. Surveillance agencies within the ministry of health perform tobacco control monitoring and regulatory, enforcement and evaluation functions.

Due to the federal structure of the country (27 states and the Federal District, with 5592 municipalities) and the decentralized nature of the health system, implementation and enforcement of most tobacco control policies are at the state and local levels. Subnational health departments and enforcement agencies constitute a powerful governmental tobacco control network with specific tobacco control focal points and devoted staff. In 2005, all states and more than two thirds of municipalities had trained staff to implement tobacco control activities, and a third of municipalities, including all major Brazilian cities, had implemented specific tobacco control programmes and enforcement actions.

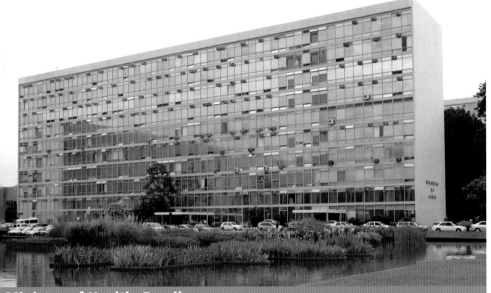

Ministry of Health, Brazil

Conclusion

The WHO Framework Convention on Tobacco Control demonstrates commitment to decisive action against the global tobacco epidemic, which kills millions of people and disables millions more each year. More than 160 Parties to the WHO FCTC, covering 86% of the world's population, have made a legally binding commitment to implement effective tobacco control policies. Unlike many leading public health problems, the means to curb tobacco use are within our reach: with the specific demand reduction measures in MPOWER and other WHO FCTC policies, countries have tobacco control tools needed to reduce tobacco use and save lives.

The results presented in this report show that progress is possible and is being made. In some countries, this progress has been rapid and sweeping – these countries can serve as models for action by countries that still need to do more to protect their people against the harms of tobacco use. If we do not continue to expand and intensify tobacco control efforts, millions of people will continue to die each year from preventable tobacco-related illness, and tens of billions of dollars will be lost annually to avoidable health-care expenditures and productivity losses.

This report shows that nearly 400 million additional people are benefiting from a tobacco control policy newly implemented during 2008 but also that there is still far more work that must be done.

- Less than 10% of the world's population is covered by any one of the MPOWER demand reduction measures.

- Progress on implementing bans on tobacco advertising, promotion and sponsorship has stalled, leaving more than 90% of the world's population without protection from tobacco industry marketing.

- Progress on increasing tobacco taxes has also come to a halt, with nearly 95% of the world's population living in countries where taxes represent less than 75% of retail price.

- Tobacco control remains severely underfunded, with 173 times as many dollars collected worldwide through tobacco tax revenues each year than are spent on tobacco control.

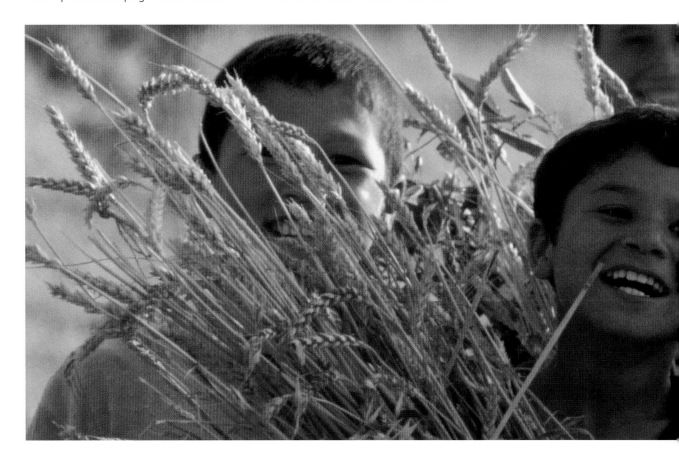

Progress has been made on smoke-free policies, which are the focus of this report, yet most people worldwide are still not protected from the dangers of second-hand tobacco smoke exposure.

- An additional 2.3% of the world's population – representing more than 154 million people – became newly covered by smoke-free laws in 2008, with nearly all living in low- and middle-income countries.

- Smoke-free policies at the subnational level are becoming increasingly common. Of the 100 biggest cities in the world, 22 are smoke-free – and three more (Rio de Janeiro, Salvador and São Paulo, all in Brazil) have become smoke-free since data for this report were collected.

- Compliance with smoke-free laws is low. Only 2% of the world's population live in countries with comprehensive smoke-free laws that also have high levels of compliance.

The current global economic crisis makes it even more imperative that countries ensure they have the means to fund effective tobacco control programmes. Increasing taxes on tobacco not only greatly reduces smoking prevalence, it also increases government revenues and generates funding that can be spent on tobacco control and other public health initiatives. However, even with existing tax rates, tobacco control remains severely underfunded, particularly among low- and middle-income countries.

Above all, in addition to funding, tobacco control requires political commitment at the highest levels of government. Unless urgent action is taken, more than 1 billion people could be killed by tobacco during this century. The success of the WHO FCTC provides strong evidence that this political will exists on national and global levels and can be tapped to great effect. By taking action to implement the measures to reduce tobacco use, governments and civil society can and will save millions of lives each year.

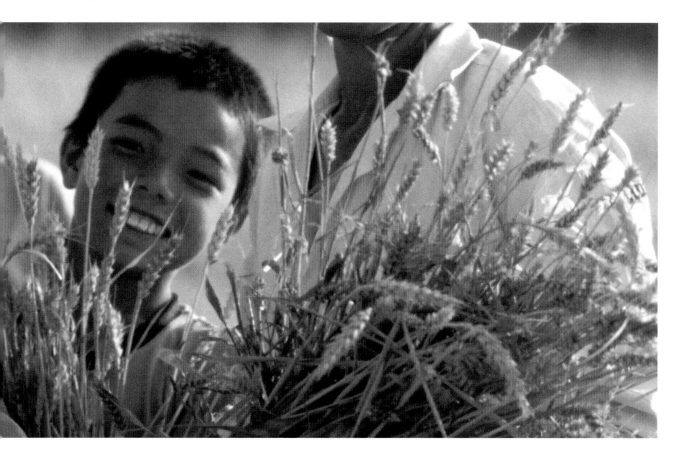

References

1. *WHO Framework Convention on Tobacco Control.* Geneva, Health Organization, 2003 (updated 2004, 2005; World http://www.who.int/tobacco/framework/WHO_FCTC_english.pdf, accessed 23 September 2009).

2. *Conference of the Parties to the WHO Framework Convention on Tobacco Control. Second session. First report of committee A.* Geneva, World Health Organization, 2007 (http://apps.who.int/gb/fctc/E/E_it2.htm, accessed 13 November 2009).

3. *WHO Framework Convention on Tobacco Control. Guidelines for implementation: Article 5.3; Article 8; Article 11; Article 13.* Geneva, World Health Organization, 2009 (http://whqlibdoc.who.int/publications/2009/9789241598224_eng.pdf, accessed 18 September 2009).

4. *Protection from exposure to second-hand tobacco smoke. Policy recommendations.* Geneva, World Health Organization, 2007 (http://whqlibdoc.who.int/publications/2007/9789241563413_eng.pdf, accessed 9 February 2009).

5. *WHO report on the global tobacco epidemic, 2008: the MPOWER package.* Geneva, World Health Organization, 2008 (http://www.who.int/tobacco/mpower/mpower_report_full_2008.pdf, accessed 13 November 2009).

6. *Tobacco smoke and involuntary smoking: summary of data reported and evaluation.* Geneva, World Health Organization, International Agency for Research on Cancer, 2002 (IARC Monographs on the Evaluation of Carcinogenic Risks to Humans, Vol. 83; http://monographs.iarc.fr/ENG/Monographs/vol83/volume83.pdf, accessed 13 November 2009).

7. Schick S, Glantz S. Philip Morris toxicological experiments with fresh sidestream smoke: more toxic than mainstream smoke. *Tobacco Control*, 2005, 14:396–404.

8. *Report on carcinogens*, 11th ed. Research Triangle Park, NC, US Department of Health and Human Services, Public Health Service, National Toxicology Program, 2005.

9. *Respiratory health effects of passive smoking.* Washington, DC, United States Environmental Protection Agency, 1992:Table 3-1.

10. Invernizzi G et al. Particulate matter from tobacco versus diesel car exhaust: an educational perspective. *Tobacco Control*, 2004, 13:219–221.

11. Singer BC et al. Gas-phase organics in environmental tobacco smoke. 1. Effects of smoking rate, ventilation, and furnishing level on emission factors. *Environmental Science and Technology*, 2002, 36:846–853.

12. Daisey JM et al. Toxic volatile organic compounds in simulated environmental tobacco smoke: emission factors for exposure assessment. *Journal of Exposure Analysis and Environmental Epidemiology*, 1998, 8:313–334.

13. Winickoff JP et al. Beliefs about the health effects of "thirdhand" smoke and home smoking bans. *Pediatrics*, 2009, 123:e74–79.

14. Navas-Acien A et al. Secondhand tobacco smoke in public places in Latin America, 2002–2003. *JAMA*, 2004, 291:2741–2745.

15. Hyland A et al. A 32-country comparison of tobacco smoke derived particle levels in indoor public places. *Tobacco Control*, 2008, 17:159–165.

16. Öberg M et al. Global estimate of the burden of disease from second-hand smoke. (unpublished).

17. *Survey on tobacco – analytical report.* Brussels, European Commission, 2009 (Flash Eurobarometer No. 253, The Gallup Organisation; http://ec.europa.eu/public_opinion/flash/fl_253_en.pdf, accessed 27 August 2009).

18. Shields M. Smoking – prevalence, bans and exposure to second-hand smoke. Ottawa, Statistics Canada, 2007. Health Reports, Vol. 18, No. 3:67–85.

19. *International Consultation on Environmental Tobacco Smoke (ETS) and Child Health.* Geneva, World Health Organization, Division of Noncommunicable Disease, Tobacco Free Initiative, 1999. (http://www.who.int/tobacco/research/en/ets_report .pdf, accessed 13 November 2009).

20. Centers for Disease Control and Prevention (CDC). Global Youth Tobacco Surveillance, 2000–2007. *Morbidity and Mortality Weekly Report*, 2007, 2008, 57: 1–21.

21. Mathers CD, Loncar D. Projections of global mortality and burden of disease from 2002 to 2030. *PLoS Medicine*, 2006, 3: e442.

22. Centers for Disease Control and Prevention (CDC). Smoking-attributable mortality, years of potential life lost, and productivity losses – United States, 2000–2004. *Morbidity and Mortality Weekly Report*, 2008, 57:1226–1228.

23. *Lifting the smokescreen: 10 reasons for a smoke free Europe.* Brussels, The Smoke Free Partnership, 2006 (http://www.ersnet.org/ers/show/default.aspx?id_attach=13509, accessed 13 April 2009).

24. Smoking and health: joint report of the Study Group on Smoking and Health. *Science*, 1957, 125:1129-1133.

25. White J, Froeb H. Small-airways dysfunction in nonsmokers chronically exposed to tobacco smoke. *New England Journal of Medicine*, 1980, 27:720–723.

26. Hirayama T. Non-smoking wives of heavy smokers have a higher risk of lung cancer: a study from Japan. *British Medical Journal*, 1981, 282:183–185.

27. Trichopoulos D et al. Lung cancer and passive smoking. *International Journal of Cancer*, 1981, 27:1–4.

28. *The health consequences of involuntary exposure to tobacco smoke: a report of the Surgeon General.* Atlanta, GA, US Department of Health and Human Services, Centers for Disease Control and Prevention, Coordinating Center for Health Promotion, National Center for Chronic Disease Prevention and Health Promotion, Office on Smoking and Health, 2006 (http://www.surgeongeneral.gov/library/secondhandsmoke/report/fullreport.pdf, accessed 13 November 2009).

29. *Proposed identification of environmental tobacco smoke as a toxic air contaminant, Scientific Review Panel approved version. Part B – Health effects.* Sacramento, CA, California Environmental Protection Agency, Office of Environmental Health Hazard Assessment, 2005 (ftp://ftp.arb.ca.gov/carbis/regact/ets2006/app3part%20b.pdf, accessed 27 August 2009).

30. *Update of evidence on health effects of secondhand smoke.* London, Scientific Committee on Tobacco and Health, 2004 (http://www.dh.gov.uk/prod_consum_dh/idcplg?IdcService=GET_FILE&dID=13632&Rendition=Web, accessed 13 November 2009).

31. Woodward A, Laugesen M. How many deaths are caused by second-hand cigarette smoke? *Tobacco Control*, 2001, 10:383–388.

32. Bridevaux PO et al. Secondhand smoke and health-related quality of life in never smokers: results from the SAPALDIA cohort study 2. *Archives of Internal Medicine*, 2007, 167:2516–2523.

33. Bertone ER et al. Environmental tobacco smoke and risk of malignant lymphoma in pet cats. *American Journal of Epidemiology*, 2002, 156:268–273.

34. Snyder LA et al. p53 expression and environmental tobacco smoke exposure in feline oral squamous cell carcinoma. *Veterinary Pathology*, 2004, 41:209–214.

35. Reif JS et al. Passive smoking and canine lung cancer risk. *American Journal of Epidemiology*, 1992, 135:234–239.

36. Fantuzzi G et al. Preterm delivery and exposure to active and passive smoking during pregnancy: a case-control study from Italy. *Paediatric and Perinatal Epidemiology*, 2007, 21:194–200.

37. Fantuzzi G et al. Exposure to active and passive smoking during pregnancy and severe small for gestational age at term. *The Journal of Maternal-fetal and Neonatal Medicine*, 2008, 21:643–647.

38. Anderson HR, Cook DG. Passive smoking and sudden infant death syndrome: review of the epidemiological evidence. *Thorax*, 1997, 52:1003–1009.

39. Law MR, Hackshaw AK. Environmental tobacco smoke. *British Medical Bulletin*, 1996, 52:22–34.

40. Gilbert SG. *Scientific consensus statement on environmental agents associated with neurodevelopmental disorders.* Bolinas, CA, Collaborative on Health and the Environment, Learning and Developmental Disabilities Initiative, 2008 (http://www.iceh.org/pdfs/LDDI/LDDIStatement.pdf, accessed 3 February 2009).

41. Herrmann M, King K, Weitzman M. Prenatal tobacco smoke and postnatal secondhand smoke exposure and child neurodevelopment. *Current Opinion in Pediatrics*, 2008, 20:184–190.

42. Behan DF et al. *Economic effects of environmental tobacco smoke.* Schaumburg, IL, Society of Actuaries, 2005 (http://www.soa.org/research/life/research-economic-effect.aspx, accessed 13 November 2009).

43. *Indoor Air Quality 1994, 59:15968-16039.* Washington, DC, United States Department of Labor, Occupational Safety and Health Administration, 1994.

44. Adams KA et al. *The costs of environmental tobacco smoke (ETS): an international review*. Geneva, World Health Organization, 1999 (WHO/NCD/TFI/99.11).

45. McGhee SM et al. Cost of tobacco-related diseases, including passive smoking, in Hong Kong. *Tobacco Control*, 2006, 15:125–130.

46. Pierce JP, León M. Effectiveness of smoke-free policies. *Lancet Oncology*, 2008, 9:614–615.

47. Haw SJ, Gruer L. Changes in exposure of adult non-smokers to secondhand smoke after implementation of smoke-free legislation in Scotland: national cross sectional survey. *British Medical Journal*, 2007, 335:549.

48. Borland R et al. Protection from environmental tobacco smoke in California. The case for a smoke-free workplace. *Journal of the American Medical Association*, 1992, 268:749–752.

49. Pickett MS et al. Smoke-free laws and secondhand smoke exposure in US non-smoking adults, 1999–2002. *Tobacco Control*, 2006, 15:302–307.

50. Mulcahy M et al. Secondhand smoke exposure and risk following the Irish smoking ban: an assessment of salivary cotinine concentrations in hotel workers and air nicotine levels in bars. *Tobacco Control*, 2005, 14:384–388.

51. Goodman P et al. Effects of the Irish smoking ban on respiratory health of bar workers and air quality in Dublin pubs. *American Journal of Respiratory and Critical Care Medicine*, 2007, 175:840–845.

52. Bondy SJ et al. Impact of an indoor smoking ban on bar workers' exposure to secondhand smoke. *Journal of Occupational and Environmental Medicine*, 2009, 51:612–619.

53. Semple S et al. Secondhand smoke levels in Scottish pubs: the effect of smoke-free legislation. *Tobacco Control*, 2007, 16:127–132.

54. Centers for Disease Control and Prevention (CDC). Reduced secondhand smoke exposure after implementation of a comprehensive statewide smoking ban, New York, June 26, 2003–June 30, 2004. *Morbidity and Mortality Weekly Report*, 2007, 56:705–708.

55. Fernando D et al. Legislation reduces exposure to second-hand tobacco smoke in New Zealand bars by about 90%. *Tobacco Control*, 2007, 16:235–238.

56. Heloma A, Jaakkola MS. Four-year follow-up of smoke exposure, attitudes and smoking behaviour following enactment of Finland's national smoke-free work-place law. *Addiction*, 2003, 98:1111–1117.

57. *Building blocks for tobacco control: a handbook*. Geneva, World Health Organization, 2004 (http://www.who.int/entity/tobacco/resources/publications/general/HANDBOOK%20Lowres%20with%20cover.pdf, accessed 13 November 2009).

58. Gan Q et al. Effectiveness of a smoke-free policy in lowering secondhand smoke concentrations in offices in China. *Journal of Occupational and Environmental Medicine*, 2008, 50:570–575.

59. Cains T et al. Designated "no smoking" areas provide from partial to no protection from environmental tobacco smoke. *Tobacco Control*, 2004, 13:17–22.

60. *Ventilation for acceptable indoor air quality*. Atlanta, GA, American Society of Heating, Refrigerating, and Air-Conditioning Engineers, Inc., 2004 (ANSI/ASHRAE Standard 62.1-2004).

61. *Environmental tobacco smoke. Position document approved by ASHRAE Board of Directors, 30 June 2005*. Atlanta, GA, American Society of Heating, Refrigerating, and Air-Conditioning Engineers, Inc., 2005.

62. *Health effects of exposure to environmental tobacco smoke*. Sacramento, CA, California Environmental Agency, Office of Environmental Health Hazard Assessment, 1997 (http://www.oehha.org/air/environmental_tobacco/finalets.html, accessed 13 November 2009).

63. *Institute for Health and Consumer Protection. Activity report 2003*. Ispra, European Commission Joint Research Centre Directorate-General, 2004 (http://ihcp.jrc.ec.europa.eu/docs/IHCP_annual_report/ihcp03.pdf, accessed 13 November 2009).

64. Valente P et al. Exposure to fine and ultrafine particles from secondhand smoke in public places before and after the smoking ban, Italy 2005. *Tobacco Control*, 2007, 16:312–3

65. Menzies D et al. Respiratory symptoms, pulmonary function, and markers of inflammation among bar workers before and after a legislative ban on smoking in public places. *Journal of the American Medical Association*, 2006, 296:1742–1748.

66. Eisner M, Smith A, Blanc P. Bartenders' respiratory health after establishment of smokefree bars and taverns. *Journal of the American Medical Association*, 1998, 280:1909–1914.

67. Venn A, Britton J. Exposure to secondhand smoke and biomarkers of cardiovascular disease risk in never-smoking adults. *Circulation*, 2007, 115:990–995.

68. Richiardi L et al. Cardiovascular benefits of smoking regulations: The effect of decreased exposure to passive smoking. *Preventive Medicine*, 2009, 48:167–172.

69. Pell JP et al. Smoke-free legislation and hospitalizations for acute coronary syndrome. *New England Journal of Medicine*, 2008, 359:482–491.

70. Bartecchi C et al. Reduction in the incidence of acute myocardial infarction associated with a citywide smoking ordinance. *Circulation*, 2006, 114:1490–1496.

71. Khuder SA et al. The impact of a smoking ban on hospital admissions for coronary heart disease. *Preventive Medicine*, 2007, 45:3–8.

72. Sargent RP et al. Reduced incidence of admissions for myocardial infarction associated with public smoking ban: before and after study. *British Medical Journal*, 2004, 328:977–980.

73. Lemstra M et al. Implications of a public smoking ban. *Canadian Journal of Public Health*, 2008, 99:62–65.

74. Meyers DG et al. Cardiovascular effect of bans on smoking in public places: a systematic review and meta-analysis. *J Am Coll Cardiol*, 2009, 29;54:1249-1255.

75. *California tobacco control update: the social norm change approach*. Sacramento, CA, California Department of Public Health, Tobacco Control Section, 2006 and 2009 (http://www.cdph.ca.gov/programs/tobacco/Pages/CTCPPublications.aspx, accessed 27 August 2009).

76. Evans W et al. Do workplace smoking bans reduce smoking? *American Economic Review*, 1999, 89:728–747.

77. Levy D, Friend K. Clean air laws: a framework for evaluating and improving clean air laws. *Journal of Public Health Management and Practice*, 2001, 7:87–97.

78. Fichtenberg CM, Glantz SA. Effect of smoke-free workplaces on smoking behaviour: systematic review. *British Medical Journal*, 2002, 325:188.

79. Bauer JE et al. A longitudinal assessment of the impact of smoke-free worksite policies on tobacco use. *American Journal of Public Health*, 2005, 95:1024–1029.

80. Fong GT et al. Reductions in tobacco smoke pollution and increases in support for smoke-free public places following the implementation of comprehensive smoke-free workplace legislation in the Republic of Ireland: findings from the International Tobacco Control (ITC) Ireland/UK Survey. *Tobacco Control*, 2006, 15(Suppl. 3):iii51–iii58.

81. Fowkes FJ et al. Scottish smoke-free legislation and trends in smoking cessation. *Addiction*, 2008, 103:1888–1895.

82. Borland RM et al. Determinants and consequences of smoke-free homes: findings from the International Tobacco Control (ITC) Four Country Survey. *Tobacco Control*, 2006, 15(Suppl. 3):iii42–iii50.

83. Wipfli H et al. Secondhand smoke exposure among women and children: evidence from 31 countries. *American Journal of Public Health* 2008, 98:672–679.

84. Borland R et al. Trends in environmental tobacco smoke restrictions in the home in Victoria, Australia. *Tobacco Control*, 1999, 8:266–271.

85. *After the smoke has cleared: evaluation of the impact of a new smokefree law*. Wellington, New Zealand Ministry of Health, 2006 (http://www.moh.govt.nz/moh.nsf/0/A9D3734516F6757ECC25723D00752D50, accessed 13 November 2009).

86. Evans D, Byrne C. *The 2004 Irish smoking ban: is there a "knock-on" effect on smoking in the home?* Dublin, Health Service Executive of the Republic of Ireland, Western Area, 2006.

87. Albers AB et al. Household smoking bans and adolescent antismoking attitudes and smoking initiation: findings from a longitudinal study of a Massachusetts youth cohort. *American Journal of Public Health*, 2008, 98:1886–1893.

88. Li Q et al. Support for smoke free policies among smokers and non-smokers in six cities in China. *Tobacco Control*, 13 August 2009 (epub ahead of print).

89. *Major new poll shows public support across UK for comprehensive smokefree law*. London, Action on Smoking and Health, Press Release 30 December 2005 (http://www.ash.org.uk/ash_jf9oyumi.htm, accessed 18 September 2009).

90. Sebrié EM et al. Smokefree environments in Latin America: on the road to real change? *Prevention and Control*, 2008, 3:21–35.

91. Equipos Mori. *Estudio de "Conocimiento y actitudes hacia el decreto 288/005" (Regulación de consumo de tabaco en lugares públicos y privados)* [*Regulation of snuff consumption in public and private places*]. Washington, DC, Organización Panamericana de la Salud (Pan American Health Organization), 2006 (http://www.presidencia.gub.uy/_web/noticias/2006/12/informeo_dec268_mori.pdf, accessed 13 November 2009).

92. *Aotearoa New Zealand smokefree workplaces: a 12-month report*. Wellington, Asthma and Respiratory Foundation of New Zealand, 2005 (http://www.no-smoke.org/pdf/NZ_TwelveMonthReport.pdf, accessed 13 November 2009).

93. *Poll shows 98% of us believe Irish workplaces are healthier as a result of the smokefree law*. Naas, Office of Tobacco Control (Press release 28 March 2005; http://www.otc.ie/article.asp?article=267, accessed 13 November 2009).

94. *California bar patrons' Field Research Corporation polls, March 1998 and September 2002*. Sacramento, CA, California Department of Public Health, Tobacco Control Section, 2002.

95. *China tobacco control report*. Beijing, Ministry of Health of the People's Republic of China, 2007.

96. Danishevski K et al. Public attitudes towards smoking and tobacco control policy in Russia. *Tobacco Control*, 2008, 17:276–283.

97. Scollo M et al. Review of the quality of studies on the economic effects of smoke-free policies on the hospitality industry. *Tobacco Control*, 2003, 12:13–20.

98. Scollo M, Lal A. *Summary of studies assessing the economic impact of smoke-free policies in the hospitality industry*. Carlton, VicHealth Centre for Tobacco Control, 2008 (http://www.vctc.org.au/downloads/Hospitalitysummary.pdf, accessed 28 August 2009).

99. Borland R et al. Support for and reported compliance with smoke-free restaurants and bars by smokers in four countries: findings from the International Tobacco Control (ITC) Four Country Survey. *Tobacco Control*, 2006, 15(Suppl. 3):iii34–iii41.

100. Lund M. Smoke-free bars and restaurants in Norway. Oslo, National Institute for Alcohol and Drug Research (SIRUS), 2005 (http://www.sirus.no/internett/tobakk/publication/375.html, accessed 13 November 2009).

101. Edwards R et al. After the smoke has cleared: evaluation of the impact of a new national smoke-free law in New Zealand. *Tobacco Control*, 2008, 17:e2.

102. Tang H et al. Changes of knowledge, attitudes, beliefs, and preference of bar owner and staff in response to a smoke-free bar law. *Tobacco Control*, 2004, 13:87–89.

103. *The state of smoke-free New York City: a one-year review*. New York: New York City Department of Finance, New York City Department of Health & Mental Hygiene, New York City Department of Small Business Services, New York City Economic Development Corporation, 2004. (http://www.nyc.gov/html/doh/downloads/pdf/smoke/sfaa-2004report.pdf, accessed 28 August 2009)

104. Eriksen M, Chaloupka F. The economic impact of clean indoor air laws. *CA: a Cancer Journal for Clinicians*, 2007, 57:367–378.

105. Hyland A, Cummings KM. Restaurant employment before and after the New York City Smoke-Free Air Act. *Journal of Public Health Management and Practice*, 1999, 5:22–27.

106. Alpert HR et al. Environmental and economic evaluation of the Massachusetts Smoke-Free Workplace Law. *Journal of Community Health*, 2007, 32:269–281.

107. Pyles MK et al. Economic effect of a smoke-free law in a tobacco-growing community. *Tobacco Control*, 2007, 16:66–68.

108. Dai C et al. *The economic impact of Florida's Smoke-Free Workplace Law*. Gainesville, FL, University of Florida, Warrington College of Business Administration, Bureau of Economic and Business Research, 2004.

109. Alamar B, Glantz SA. Effect of smoke-free laws on bar value and profits. *American Journal of Public Health*, 2007, 97:1400–1402.

110. Binkin N et al. Effects of a generalised ban on smoking in bars and restaurants, Italy. *International Journal of Tuberculosis and Lung Disease*, 2007, 11:522–527.

111. *A study of public attitudes toward cigarette smoking and the tobacco industry in 1978*, Vol. 1. Storrs: The Roper Organization, 1978 (http://legacy.library.ucsf.edu/tid/qra99d00/pdf, accessed 13 November 2009).

112. Heironimus J. *Impact of workplace restrictions on consumption and incidence*. Tobacco Documents Online, 1992 (http:// tobaccodocuments.org/pm/2023914280-4284.html, accessed 13 November 2009).

113. Sebrie E, Glantz S. "Accommodating" smoke-free policies: tobacco industry's Courtesy of Choice programme in Latin America. *Tobacco Control*, 2007, 16:e6.

114. *Smoking in public places. House of Commons Health Committee, first report of session 2005–2006, Vol. II*. London, House of Commons, 2005 (http://www.publications. parliament.uk/pa/cm200506/cmselect/cmhealth/485/485ii.pdf, accessed 13 November 2009).

115. Samet JM, Burke TA. Turning science into junk: the tobacco industry and passive smoking. *American Journal of Public Health*, 2001, 91:1742–1744.

116. Ong EK, Glantz SA. Tobacco industry efforts subverting International Agency for Research on Cancer's second-hand smoke study. *Lancet*, 2000, 355:1253–1259.

117. Ong EK, Glantz SA. Constructing "sound science" and "good epidemiology": tobacco, lawyers, and public relations firms. *American Journal of Public Health*, 2001, 91:1749–1757.

118. Tong EK, Glantz SA. Tobacco industry efforts undermining evidence linking secondhand smoke with cardiovascular disease. *Circulation*, 2007, 116:1845–1854.

119. Bornhauser A et al. German tobacco industry's successful efforts to maintain scientific and political respectability prevent regulation of secondhand smoke. *Tobacco Control*, 2006, 15:e1.

120. Robinson JB. *ETS in Nordic countries*. Paper presented at PM EEC ETS Conference, Geneva, 12–14 November 198, San Francisco, CA, University of California Legacy Tobac Documents Library, 1986.

121. Tobacco Institute. *Embargoed for use in A.M. newspape, Monday 810615*. San Francisco, CA, University of Califor Legacy Tobacco Documents Library, 1981 (Philip Morris Collection; Bates No. 2015018011/8012; http://legacy. library.ucsf.edu/tid/arl68e00, accessed 13 November 20

122. Barnes DE, Bero LA. Why review articles on the health effects of passive smoking reach different conclusions. *Journal of the American Medical Association*, 1998, 279:1566–1570.

123. Barnes DE, Bero LA. Scientific quality of original researc articles on environmental tobacco smoke. *Tobacco Cont*, 1997, 6:19–26.

124. Garne D et al. Environmental tobacco smoke research published in the journal Indoor and Built Environment and associations with the tobacco industry. *Lancet*, 200 365:804–809.

125. United States of America v. Philip Morris USA, Inc., et al, 449 F Supp 2d 1 (2006).

126. Siegel M. The effectiveness of state-level tobacco contro interventions: a review of program implementation and behavioral outcomes. *Annual Review of Public Health*, 2002, 23:45–71.

127. Jones JM. *Smoking habits stable; most would like to qui*, Washington: Gallup, Inc., 2006. (http://www.gallup.com poll/23791/Smoking-Habits-Stable-Most-Would-Like-Qu aspx, accessed 13 November 2009).

128. Fiore MC et al. Treating tobacco use and dependence: 2008 update. Clinical practice guideline. Rockville, MD, Department of Health and Human Services, Public Healt Service, 2008 (http://www.surgeongeneral.gov/tobacco, treating_tobacco_use08.pdf, accessed 13 November 20

129. Conference of the Parties to the WHO Framework Convention on Tobacco Control. Third session. Decisions Geneva, World Health Organization, 2008 (http://apps.v int/gb/fctc/PDF/cop3/FCTC_COP3_DIV3-en.pdf, accessed 13 November 2009).

130. Cromwell J et al. Cost-effectiveness of the clinical pract recommendations in the AHCPR guideline for smoking cessation. Agency for Health Care Policy and Research. *Journal of the American Medical Association*, 1997, 278:1759–1766.

131. Doll R et al. Mortality in relation to smoking: 50 years' observations on male British doctors. *British Medical Journal*, 2004, 328(7455):1519–1527.

132. *The health benefits of smoking cessation: a report of the Surgeon General*. Rockville, MD, US Department of Heal and Human Services. Centers for Disease Control, Cente for Chronic Disease Prevention and Health Promotion, Office on Smoking and Health, 1990 (HYPERLINK "http: profiles.nlm.nih.gov/NN/B//C/T/_/nnbbct.pdf"http:// profiles.nlm.nih.gov/NN/B/B/C/T/_/nnbbct.pdf, accessed September 2009).

133. *Everybody's business – Strengthening health systems to improve health outcomes: WHO's framework for action*. Geneva, World Health Organization, 2007 (http://www.searo.who.int/LinkFiles/Health_Systems_ EverybodyBusinessHSS.pdf, accessed 13 November 200

134. *WHO CVD-risk management package for low- and medi resource settings*. Geneva, World Health Organization, 2 (http://whqlibdoc.who.int/publications/2002/92415458 pdf, accessed 13 November 2009).

135. *WHO/The Union monograph on TB and tobacco control: joining efforts to control two related global epidemics.* Geneva, World Health Organization, 2007 (http://www.who.int/tobacco/resources/publications/tb_tobac_monograph.pdf, accessed 13 November 2009).

136. Stead LF et al. A systematic review of interventions for smokers who contact quitlines. *Tobacco Control*, 2007, 16(Suppl. 1):i13–i18.

137. *WHO Model List of Essential Medicines: 16th list, March 2009.* Geneva, World Health Organization, 2009 (Unedited version – 30 April 2009) (http://www.who.int/selection_medicines/committees/expert/17/WEB_unedited_16th_LIST.pdf, accessed 20 October 2009).

138. Hammond D et al. Effectiveness of cigarette warning labels in informing smokers about the risks of smoking: findings from the International Tobacco Control (ITC) Four Country Survey. *Tobacco Control*, 2006, 15(Suppl. 3):iii19–iii25.

139. *Youth and tobacco: Preventing tobacco use among young people.* A report of the Surgeon General. Rockville, MD, US Department of Health and Human Services. Centers for Disease Control and Prevention, National Center for Chronic Disease Prevention and Health Promotion, Office on Smoking and Health, 1994.

140. *Elaboration of guidelines for implementation: Articles 5.3, 9 and 10, 11, 12 and 14 (decision FCTC/COP2(14).* Geneva, World Health Organization, Conference of the Parties to the WHO Framework Convention on Tobacco Control. 2007 (http://apps.who.int/gb/fctc/PDF/cop2/FCTC_COP2_DIV9-en.pdf, accessed 18 September 2009).

141. Datafolha Instituto de Pesquisas. 76% são a favor que embalagens de cigarros tragam imagens que ilustram males provocados pelo fumo; 67% dos fumantes que viram as imagens afirmam terem sentido vontade de parar de fumar. [76% are in favor of pictures on cigarette packs that illustrate the problems caused by smoking, 67% of smokers saw the pictures and say they made them want to stop smoking] *Opinião pública*, 2002.

142. *Tobacco warning labels.* Geneva, Framework Convention Alliance for Tobacco Control, 2005 (Factsheet No. 7; http://tobaccofreekids.org/campaign/global/docs/7.pdf, accessed 13 November 2009).

143. Thrasher JF et al. Smokers' reactions to cigarette package warnings with graphic imagery and with only text: a comparison between Mexico and Canada. *Salud Pública de México*, 2007, 49 (Suppl. 2):S233–S240.

144. *Up in smoke: the truth about tar and nicotine ratings.* Washington, DC, Federal Trade Commission, Bureau of Consumer Protection, Office of Consumer and Business Education, 2000 (FTC Consumer Alert; http://www.ftc.gov/bcp/edu/pubs/consumer/alerts/alt069.shtm, accessed 13 November 2009).

145. Siegel M, Biener L. The impact of an antismoking media campaign on progression to established smoking: results of a longitudinal youth study. *American Journal of Public Health*, 2000, 90:380–386.

146. McVey D, Stapleton J. Can anti-smoking television advertising affect smoking behaviour? Controlled trial of the Health Education Authority for England's anti-smoking TV campaign. *Tobacco Control*, 2000, 9:273–282.

147. Dunlop SM et al. The contribution of antismoking advertising to quitting: intra- and interpersonal processes. *Journal of Health Communication*, 2008;13:250–266.

148. Wakefield M et al. Effect of televised, tobacco company-funded smoking prevention advertising on youth smoking-related beliefs, intentions, and behavior. *American Journal of Public Health*, 2006, 96:2154–2160.

149. *American Cancer Society/UICC Tobacco Control Strategy Planning Guide #4. Enforcing Strong Smoke-free Laws: The Advocate's Guide to Enforcement Strategies.* Atlanta, American Cancer Society, 2006.

150. *Cigarette report for 2003.* Washington, DC, Federal Trade Commission, 2005 (http://www.ftc.gov/reports/cigarette05/050809cigrpt.pdf, accessed 13 November 2009).

151. Saffer H, Chaloupka F. The effect of tobacco advertising bans on tobacco consumption. *Journal of Health Economics*, 2000, 19:1117–1137.

152. Jha P, Chaloupka FJ, eds. *Curbing the epidemic: governments and the economics of tobacco control.* Washington, DC, The World Bank, 1999 (http://www.usaid.gov/policy/ads/200/tobacco.pdf, accessed 13 November 2009).

153. Crofton J, Simpson D. *Tobacco: a global threat.* Hong Kong, Macmillan Education, 2002.

154. *Select Committee on Health, second report.* London, House of Commons, 2000 (http://www.parliament.the-stationery-office.co.uk/pa/cm199900/cmselect/cmhealth/27/2702.htm, accessed 13 November 2009).

155. Jha P et al. Tobacco addiction. In: Jamison D et al., eds. *Disease control priorities in developing countries*, 2nd ed. Washington, DC, The World Bank, 2006:869–885 (http://files.dcp2.org/pdf/DCP/DCP46.pdf, accessed 13 November 2009).

156. van Walbeek C. *Tobacco excise taxation in South Africa.* Geneva, World Health Organization, 2003 (http://www.who.int/tobacco/training/success_stories/en/best_practices_south_africa_taxation.pdf, accessed 13 November 2009).

157. Centers for Disease Control and Prevention (CDC). Response to increases in cigarette prices by race/ethnicity, income, and age groups – United States, 1976–1993. *Morbidity and Mortality Weekly Report*, 1998, 47:605–609.

158. Chaloupka FJ et al. The taxation of tobacco products. In: Jha P, Chaloupka FJ, eds. *Tobacco control in developing countries.* New York, Oxford University Press, 2000:2737–2772.

159. Joossens L. *Report on smuggling control in Spain.* Geneva, World Health Organization, 2003 (http://www.who.int/tobacco/training/success_stories/en/best_practices_spain_smuggling_control.pdf, accessed 13 November 2009).

160. *Third session of the Intergovernmental Negotiating Body on a Protocol on Illicit Trade in Tobacco Products.* Geneva, World Health Organization, Conference of the Parties to the WHO Framework Convention on Tobacco Control, 2009 (http://www.who.int/fctc/inb/third_session_inb/en/index.html, accessed 20 October 2009).

161. Data provided by the National Statistics Office and the Excise Department, Thailand. Analyzed by B. Sarunya and T. Lakkhana, Tobacco Control Research and Knowledge Management Center (TRC), Mahidol University, 2007.

162. *Demographic Yearbook: Table 8. Population of capital cities and cities of 100 000 and more inhabitants, latest available year: 1988-2007.* New York, United Nations, United Nations Statistics Division, 2009 (http://unstats.un.org/unsd/Demographic/Products/dyb/dyb2007.htm, accessed 3 November 2009).

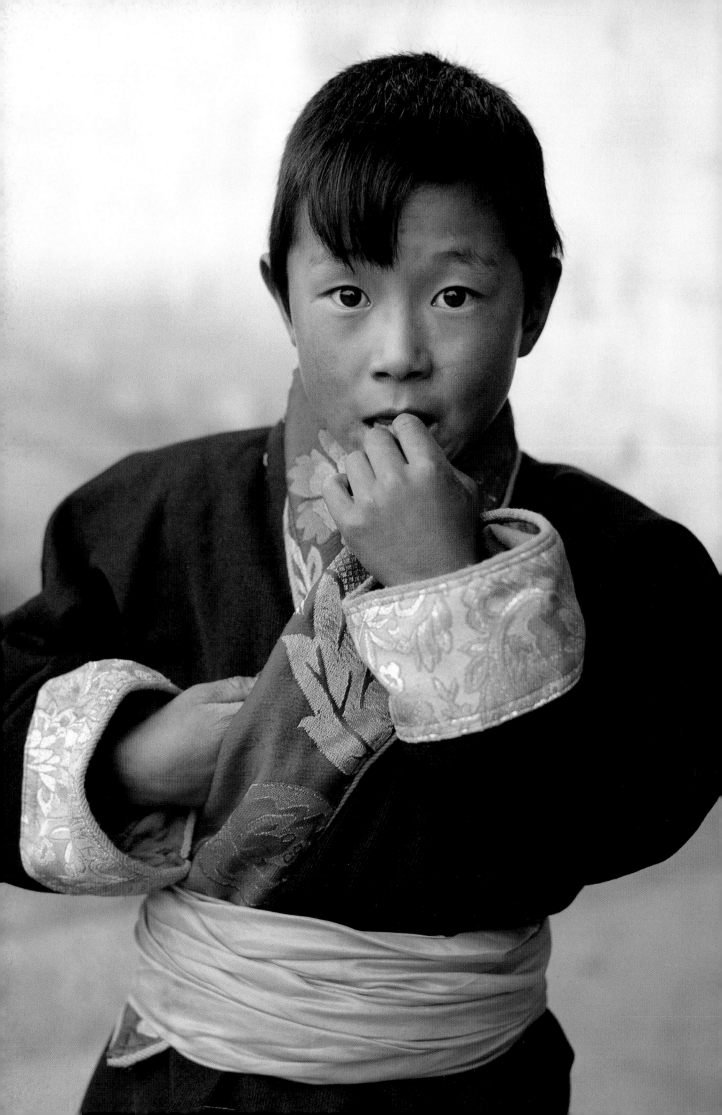

reflect the additional information collected on the survey periodicity. Periodicity of surveys of at least every five years is included in the highest category in addition to the requirements of recent and representative data for adults and youth. Because of this, some countries that fell in the highest category in the first report (defined as those having recent and representative data only) do not fall in the highest category in this second report. The groupings for the Monitoring indicator are listed below.

	No known data or no recent* data or data that are not both recent* and not representative**
	Recent* and representative** data for either adults or youth
	Recent* and representative** data for both adults and youth
	Recent*, representative** and periodic*** data for both adults and youth

*   Data from 2003 or later.
**   Survey sample representative of the national population.
***   Occurring at least every five years.

Smoke-free legislation

There is a wide range of places and institutions where it is possible to prohibit smoking. Smoke-free legislation can take place at the national or subnational level. This year's report includes items to measure national legislation as well as legislation in subnational jurisdictions. The assessment of subnational smoke-free legislation includes large jurisdictions that are first-level administrative boundaries (first administrative subdivisions of a country) and, in addition, large cities with over 5 million inhabitants or encompassing more than 20% of the country's population.

This year's questionnaire included items measuring whether smoke-free laws existed in each of the following places at either the national or subnational level:
- health-care facilities;
- educational facilities other than universities;
- universities;
- government facilities;
- indoor offices;
- restaurants;
- pubs and bars;
- public transport.

For this year's report, groupings for the Smoke-free Legislation indicator have been revised so that they are based on the numbers of places and institutions where smoking is completely prohibited. In addition, countries where at least 90% of the population are covered by complete subnational smoke-free legislation are grouped in the top category. Subnational smoke-free legislation is considered "comprehensive" when smoking in all of the public places assessed is completely banned.

In several countries, in order to significantly expand the creation of smoke-free places, including restaurants and bars, it was politically necessary to include exceptions to the law that allowed for the provision of designated smoking rooms. The requirements for designated smoking rooms are so technically complex and stringent that, for practical purposes, few or no establishments are expected to implement them. Because no data were requested on the number of complex designated smoking rooms actually constructed, it is not possible to know whether these laws have resulted in the complete absence of such rooms,

as intended. For this reason, these few countries have not been categorized in the analyses for this section.

The groupings for the Smoke-free Legislation indicator are listed below.

	Data not reported/not categorized
	Up to two public places completely smoke-free
	Three to five public places completely smoke-free
	Six to seven public places completely smoke-free
	All public places completely smoke-free (or at least 90% of the population covered by complete subnational smoke-free legislation)

Future data collection efforts will include such measures, as well as incorporate evaluation of legislation enforcement. As noted at the beginning of this report, as well as in the WHO FCTC Article 8 guidelines and several other governmental and nongovernmental reports, ventilation and other forms of designated smoking areas do not fully protect from the harms of second-hand tobacco smoke, and the only laws that provide complete protection are those that result in the complete absence of smoking in all public places.

Tobacco dependence treatment

Despite the low cost of quit lines, few low- or middle-income countries have implemented such programmes. Thus, national toll-free quit lines are included as a qualification only for the highest category. Reimbursement for tobacco dependence treatment is considered only for the top two categories, to take the tight national budgets of many lower-income countries into consideration.

The top three categories reflect varying levels of government commitment to the availability of nicotine replacement therapy and cessation support. The groupings for the Tobacco Dependence Treatment indicator are listed below.

	Data not reported
	None
	NRT* and/or some cessation services** (neither cost-covered)
	NRT* and/or some cessation services** (at least one of which is cost-covered)
	National quit line, and both NRT* and some cessation services** cost-covered

*   Nicotine replacement therapy.
** Smoking cessation support available in any of the following places: health clinics or other primary care facilities, hospitals, office of a health professional, the community.

Health warnings

The section of the questionnaire devoted to measuring health warnings asked the data collector to note the following information about the cigarette pack warnings:

- the mandated size of the warnings, as a percentage of the front and back of the cigarette pack;
- whether specific health warnings are mandated;
- whether the warnings appear on individual packages as well as on any outside packaging and labelling used in retail sale;
- whether the warnings describe specific harmful effects of tobacco use on health;
- whether the warnings are large, clear, visible and legible (e.g. specific colours and font style and sizes are mandated);
- whether the warnings rotate;
- whether the warnings are written in (all) principal language(s) of the country.

The size of the warning on front and back of the cigarette pack was averaged

to calculate the percentage of the total pack surface area that is covered by the warnings. This information was combined with the warning characteristics to construct the groupings for the Health Warnings indicator. The groupings for the Health Warnings indicator are listed below.

	Data not reported
	No warning or warning covering <30% of pack surface
	≥30%* but no pictures or pictograms and/or other appropriate characteristics**
	31%–49%* including pictures or pictograms and other appropriate characteristics**
	≥50%* including pictures or pictograms and appropriate characteristics**

*   average of the front and back of the cigarette pack.
** • Specific health warnings mandated;
     • appearing on individual packages as well as on any outside packaging and labelling used in retail sale;
     • describing specific harmful effects of tobacco use on health;
     • are large, clear, visible and legible (e.g. specific colours and font style and sizes are mandated);
     • rotate;
     • written in (all) principal language(s) of the country.

Bans on advertising, promotion and sponsorship

The section of the questionnaire devoted to measuring bans on advertising, promotion and sponsorship asked the data collector to note whether advertising bans covered the following types of advertising:

- national television and radio;
- local magazines and newspapers;
- billboards and outdoor advertising;
- point of sale;
- free distribution of tobacco products in the mail or through other means;
- promotional discounts;
- non-tobacco products identified with tobacco brand names (brand extension);
- brand names of non-tobacco products used for tobacco products;

- appearance of tobacco products in television and/or films;
- sponsored events.

The first four bans listed are considered "direct" advertising bans, and the remaining six are considered "indirect" bans. Complete bans on tobacco advertising, promotion and sponsorship usually start with bans on direct advertising in national media and progress to bans on indirect advertising as well as promotion and sponsorship. Bans that cover national TV, radio and print media were used as the basic criteria for the two lowest groups, and the remaining groups were constructed based on how comprehensively the law covers the forms of direct and indirect bans included in the questionnaire.

The groupings for the Bans on Advertising, Promotion and Sponsorship indicator are listed below.

	Data not reported
	Complete absence of ban, or ban that does not cover national television (TV), radio and print media
	Ban on national TV, radio and print media only
	Ban on national TV, radio and print media as well as on some but not all other forms of direct* and/or indirect** advertising
	Ban on all forms of direct* and indirect** advertising

*   Direct advertising bans:
     • national television and radio;
     • local magazines and newspapers;
     • billboards and outdoor advertising;
     • point of sale.
** Indirect advertising bans:
     • free distribution of tobacco products in the mail or through other means;
     • promotional discounts;
     • non-tobacco products identified with tobacco brand names (brand extension);
     • brand names of non-tobacco products used for tobacco products;
     • appearance of tobacco products in television and/or films;
     • sponsored events.

Tobacco tax levels

Countries are grouped according to the percentage contribution of taxes to the retail price. Taxes assessed include excise tax, value added tax (sometimes called "VAT"), import duty (when the cigarettes were imported) and any other taxes levied. Only the price of the most popular brand of cigarettes is considered. In the case of countries where different levels of taxes applied to cigarettes are based on either length, quantity produced or type (e.g. filter vs. non-filter), only the rate that applied to the most popular brand is used in the calculation.

Given the lack of information on country- and brand-specific profit margins of retailers and wholesalers, their profits were assumed to be zero (unless provided by the national data collector). The groupings for the Tobacco Tax indicator are listed below.

	Data not reported
	≤ 25% of retail price is tax
	26–50% of retail price is tax
	51–75% of retail price is tax
	>75% of retail price is tax

National tobacco control programmes

Classification of countries' national tobacco control programmes is based on the existence of a national agency with responsibility for tobacco control objectives as a minimum criterion for group 3. Countries with at least 5 full-time equivalent staff members working at the national agency with responsibility for tobacco control meet the criteria for the highest group.

The groupings for the National Tobacco Control Programme indicator are listed below.

	Data not reported
	No national agency or no national objectives on tobacco control
	Existence of national agency with responsibility for tobacco control objectives with no or < 5 full-time equivalent staff members
	Existence of national agency with responsibility for tobacco control objectives and at least 5 full-time equivalent staff members

Compliance assessment

Compliance with national and comprehensive subnational smoke-free legislation as well as with advertising, promotion and sponsorship bans (covering both direct and indirect marketing) was assessed by a group of five national experts, who assessed the compliance in these two areas as "minimal", "moderate" or "high". These five experts were selected by the national data collector according to the following criteria:

- person in charge of tobacco prevention in the country's ministry of health, or the most senior government official in charge of tobacco control or tobacco-related conditions;
- the head of a prominent nongovernmental organization dedicated to tobacco control;
- a health professional (e.g. physician, nurse, pharmacist or dentist) specializing in tobacco-related conditions;
- a staff member of a public health university department;
- the Tobacco Free Initiative focal point of the WHO country office.

The experts performed their assessments independently through an interview with the national data collector. Summary scores were calculated by WHO from the five individual assessments by assigning two points for highly enforced policies, one point for moderately enforced policies and no point for minimally enforced policies, with a potential minimum of 0 and maximum of 10 points in total from these five experts.

The country-reported answers to each survey question are listed in Appendix IV. Appendix I summarizes this information. Compliance scores are represented separately (i.e. compliance is not included in the calculation of the grouping categories). As noted above, future data collection efforts will include a more extensive assessment of legislation enforcement, and this assessment will be used to construct the categories of MPOWER measures.

[1] Parties report on the implementation of the WHO Framework Convention on Tobacco Control according to Article 21. The objective of reporting is to enable Parties to learn from each other's experience in implementing the WHO FCTC. Parties' reports are also the basis for review by the COP of the implementation of the Convention. Parties submit their initial report two years after entry into force of the WHO FCTC for that Party, and then every subsequent three years, through the reporting instrument adopted by COP. For more information please refer to http://www.who.int/fctc/reporting/en/.

Smoking prevalence in WHO Member States

Monitoring the prevalence of tobacco use is central to any surveillance system involved with tobacco control. Reliable prevalence data provide the information needed to assess the impacts of tobacco control actions adopted by a country and can be used by tobacco control workers in their efforts to counter the tobacco epidemic. This report contains prevalence estimates for smoking for 145 countries (see Appendix VII).

Collection of tobacco use prevalence estimates

As discussed in Technical Note I, the data collection questionnaire for this report included a detailed section on surveys of tobacco use. The section on Monitoring in Technical Note I provides a full discussion of information that was submitted by countries regarding their existing surveys of tobacco use. Data were requested on four indicators of tobacco smoking:

- current and daily prevalence of tobacco smoking; [1]
- current and daily prevalence of cigarette smoking.

These indicators provide for the most complete representation of tobacco smoking across countries and at the same time help to minimize attrition of countries from further analysis due to lack of adequate data. Although we realize that differences exist in the types of tobacco products used in different countries and grown or manufactured in different regions of the world, data on cigarette smoking and tobacco smoking are the most widely available and are common to all countries, thereby permitting statistical analyses. [2]

The information collected from countries about their recent surveys of tobacco use was checked against WHO's Global Infobase, a portal of information on eight

risk factors for noncommunicable diseases including tobacco (www.who.int/infobase). This enabled both validation of data already held by WHO as well as permitted an updating of the Global Infobase. In addition, an extensive literature search was conducted to try and identify any other possible data sources.

During this process, multiple data sources were frequently identified. In such cases, preference was given to surveys that met the following four criteria:

- provide country survey summary data for one or more of four tobacco use definitions: daily smoker, current smoker, daily cigarette smoker, or current cigarette smoker;
- include randomly selected participants who were representative of a general population;
- present prevalence values by age and sex;
- survey the adult population aged 15 years and above.

Data identified from new collections identified through the questionnaires and literature searches were entered into the Global Infobase.

Analysis and presentation of tobacco use prevalence estimates

Data collected on prevalence estimates are presented in this report in two forms:

1. Crude prevalence rates (Appendix VIII): these should be used to assess the actual use of tobacco in a country and to generate an estimate of the number of smokers for the relevant indicator (e.g. current smokers, daily smokers) in the population.

2. Adjusted and age-standardized prevalence rates (Appendix VII): these rates are constructed solely for the purpose of comparing tobacco use prevalence

estimates across multiple countries or across multiple time periods for the same country. These rates should not be used to estimate the number of smokers in the population. The methods for adjusting and age-standardizing for survey differences are described separately below, but the estimates presented in Appendix VII have been both adjusted and age standardized.

Crude prevalence. The crude smoking prevalence, a summary measure of tobacco use in a population, reflects the actual use of tobacco in a country (e.g. prevalence of smoking by adults aged 15 years and above). The crude rate, expressed as a percentage of the total population, refers to the number of smokers per 100 population of the country. When this crude prevalence rate is multiplied by the country's population, the result is the number of smokers in the country.

Adjusted prevalence. Adjustments to data are typically done when collecting information from heterogeneous sources that originate from different surveys and do not employ standardized survey instruments. These differences render difficult the production of national-level age-standardized rates. WHO has also developed a regression method that attempts to adjust the estimates to enable comparisons of the results between countries. The general principal that underlies the regression method is that if data are partly missing or are incomplete for a country, then the regression technique uses data available for the region in which the country is located to generate estimates for that country. The regression models are run at the United Nations sub-regional level [3] separately for males and females in order to obtain age-specific prevalence rates for that region. These estimates are then substituted for the country falling within the sub-region for the missing indicator. Note that the technique cannot be used for countries without any data: these countries are excluded from any analysis. The four types of differences between surveys and the relevant adjustment procedures used are listed below.

Differences in age groups covered by the survey. In order to estimate smoking prevalence rates for standard age ranges (by five-year groups from age 15 until age 80 and thereafter from 80 to 100 years), the association between age and daily smoking is examined for males and females separately for each country using scatter plots. For this exercise, data from the latest nationally representative survey are chosen; in some cases more than one survey is chosen if male and female prevalence rates stem from different surveys or if the additional survey supplements data for the extreme age intervals. To obtain age-specific prevalence rates for five-year age intervals, regression models using daily smoking prevalence estimates from a first order, second order and third order function of age are graphed against the scatter plot and the best fitting curve is chosen. For the remaining indicators, a combination of methods is applied: regression models are run at the sub-regional level to obtain age-specific rates for current and daily cigarette smoking, and an equivalence relationship is applied between smoking prevalence rates and cigarette smoking where cigarette smoking is dominant to obtain age-specific prevalence rates for current and daily cigarette smoking for the standard age intervals.

Differences in the types of indicators of tobacco use measured. If we have data for current tobacco smoking and current cigarette smoking, then definitional adjustments are made to account for the missing daily tobacco smoking and daily cigarette smoking. Likewise, if we have data for current and daily tobacco smoking only, then tobacco type adjustments are made across tobacco types to generate estimates for current and daily cigarette smoking.

Differences in geographic coverage of the survey within the country. Adjustments are made to the data by observing the prevalence relationship between urban and rural areas in countries falling within the relevant sub-region. Results from this urban-rural regression exercise are applied to countries to allow a scaling-up of prevalence to the national level. As an

example, if a country has prevalence rates for daily smoking of tobacco in urban areas only, the regression results from the rural-urban smoking relationship are used to obtain rural prevalence rates for daily smoking. These are then combined with urban prevalence rates using urban-rural population ratios as weights to generate a national prevalence estimate as well as national age-specific rates.

Differences in survey year. For this report, smoking prevalence estimates are generated for year 2006. Smoking prevalence data are sourced from surveys conducted in countries in different years. In some cases, the latest available prevalence data came from surveys before the year 2006 while in other cases the survey was later than 2006. To obtain smoking prevalence estimates for 2006, trend information is used either to project into the future for countries with data older than 2006 or backtracked for countries with data later than 2006. This is achieved by incorporating trend information from all available surveys for each country. For countries without historical data, trend information from the respective sub-region in which they fall is used.

In the absence of crude prevalence rates for the relevant indicator, adjusted prevalence estimates can be used to assess the number of smokers for the relevant indicator in a country.

Age-standardized prevalence. Tobacco use generally varies widely by sex and across age groups. Although the crude prevalence rate is reasonably easy to understand for a country at one point in time, comparing crude rates between two or more countries at one point in time, or of one country at different points in time, can be misleading if the two populations being compared have significantly different age distributions or differences in tobacco use by sex. The method of age-standardization is commonly used to overcome this problem and allows for meaningful comparison of prevalence between countries. The method involves applying the age-specific

rates by sex in each population to one standard population. When presenting age-standardized prevalence rates, both this and the WHO Report on the Global Tobacco Epidemic, 2008 used the WHO Standard Population, a fictitious population whose age distribution was artificially created and is largely reflective of the population age structure of low- and middle-income countries. The resulting age-standardized rate, also expressed as a percentage of the total population, refers to the number of smokers per 100 WHO Standard Population. As a result, the rate generated using this process is only a hypothetical number with no inherent meaning in its magnitude. It is only useful when contrasting rates obtained from one country to those obtained in another country, or from the same country at a different points in time. In order to produce an overall smoking prevalence rate for a country, the age-standardized prevalence rates for males and females must be combined to generate total prevalence. Since the WHO Standard Population is the same irrespective of sex, the age-standardized rates for males and females are combined using population weights for males and for females at the global level from the UN population data for 2006. For example, if the age-standardized prevalence rate for tobacco smoking in adults is 60% for males and 30% for females, the combined prevalence rate for tobacco smoking in all adults is calculated as 60 x (0.51) + 30 x (0.49) = 45%, with the figures in brackets representing male and female population weights. Thus, of the total smoking prevalence (45%) the proportion of smoking attributable to males is 66.7% [= (30 ÷ 45) x 100] and to females 33.3% [= (15 ÷ 45) x 100]. These combined rates are shown in Appendix VII.

[1] Tobacco smoking includes cigarettes, cigars, pipes and any other form of smoked tobacco.
[2] For countries where consumption of smokeless tobacco products is high, we have published these data for that particular country.
[3] There are 21 United Nations sub-regions; Oceania, Melanesia, Polynesia and Micronesia are combined into one subregion to form a total of 18. For a complete listing, please refer to World Population Prospects, 2008 Revision at http://esa.un.org/unpp/index.asp?panel=5 (accessed 29 September 2009).

Tobacco taxes in WHO Member States

This report includes appendices containing information on the share of total and excise taxes in the price of the most widely sold brand of cigarettes, based on tax policy information collected from each country. As described below, the figures were calculated by WHO based on submitted data. Because of these calculations, the figures published in this report may differ from those submitted by country data collectors. This note contains information on the methodology used by WHO to calculate the share of total and tobacco excise taxes in the price of a cigarette pack for this report using country-reported data.

Data collection

As discussed in Technical Note I, the data collection questionnaire for this report included a detailed section on the taxation of tobacco products in each country, as well as any supporting documents such as laws, decrees, or other official materials.

Not all taxes increase the price of tobacco. For example, taxes on the profits of tobacco manufacturers have no impact on price. Other features of tax systems, such as tax credits and amortization policies, generally have no impact either and are very difficult to analyse. For this reason, the data requested in the questionnaire focus on the types of taxes that usually have a direct impact on price.

Indirect taxes include various types of excise taxes, import duties and value added-taxes. The most important of these taxes, however, are excise taxes, because they are applied specifically to tobacco and are responsible for substantially increasing the price of tobacco products. Thus, the rates, amounts, functioning and application of excise taxes are central components of the data being collected and are an important tool in reducing tobacco consumption.

The table below describes the types of tax information collected:

1. Amount-specific excise taxes	An amount-specific excise tax is a tax *on a selected good* produced for sale within a country, or imported and sold in that country. In general, the tax is collected from the manufacturer/wholesaler or at the point of entry into the country by the importer, in addition to import duties. These taxes come in the form of an amount per pack, per 1000 sticks, or per kilogram. Example: US$ 1.50 per pack of 20 cigarettes.
2. Ad valorem excise taxes	An ad valorem excise tax is a tax *on a selected good* produced for sale within a country, or imported and sold in that country. In general, the tax is collected from the manufacturer/wholesaler or at the point of entry into the country by the importer, in addition to import duties. These taxes come in the form of a percentage of the value of a transaction between two independent entities at some point of the production/distribution chain; ad valorem taxes are generally applied to the value of the transactions between the manufacturer and the retailer/wholesaler. Example: 27% of the retail price.
3. Tobacco-specific import duties	An import duty is a tax *on a selected good* imported into a country to be consumed in that country (i.e. the goods are not in transit to another country). In general, the import duties are collected from the importer at the point of entry into the country. These taxes can be either amount-specific or ad valorem. Amount-specific import duties are applied in the same fashion as amount-specific excise taxes. Ad valorem import duties are generally applied to the CIF (cost, insurance, freight) value (i.e. the value of the unloaded consignment that includes the cost of the product itself, insurance and transport and unloading). Example: 50% import duty levied on CIF.
4. Value added taxes	The value added tax (VAT) is a "multi-stage" tax *on all consumer goods and services* applied proportionally to the price the consumer pays for a product. Although manufacturers and wholesalers also participate in the administration and payment of the tax all along the manufacturing/distribution chain, they are all reimbursed through a tax credit system, so that the only person who pays in the end is the final consumer. Most countries that impose a VAT do so on a base that includes any excise tax and customs duty. Example: VAT representing 10% of the retail price.
5. Other taxes	Any other tax that is not called an excise tax or VAT but applies to either the quantity of tobacco or to the value of a transaction of tobacco product was reported in the questionnaire, with as much detail as possible regarding what is taxed (base), who pays the tax and how the base is taxed.

The data reported in the questionnaires were provided through contacts with the ministries of finance. Where possible, the information was again checked against supporting documents. The nature of the supporting documents for tobacco taxation was in most cases laws or decrees, but other sources were used depending on the legal structure of the country. Secondary sources were also used if any doubts remained, and most of the information was actually downloaded from ministry of finance web sites. In the case of imported cigarettes, import data was used from the United Nations Comtrade database web site (http://comtrade.un.org/db/).

Data analysis

Only the price of the most widely sold brand of cigarettes was considered. In the case of countries where different levels of taxes are applied to cigarettes based on either length of cigarette, quantity produced or type (e.g. filter vs. non-filter), only the rate that applied to the most widely sold brand was used in the calculation. The only exceptions were made in Canada and the United States where, in addition to federal taxes, state/provincial taxes are applied. Therefore, an average price and average state/provincial tax were calculated in order to estimate the total tax rate of a pack of cigarettes.

The import duty was only applied to most popular brand of cigarettes that were imported into the country. Countries which reported that the most popular brand was produced locally were not imposed an import duty.

Excise taxes and VAT were applied wherever existent and applicable in the country.

"Other taxes" are all other taxes excluding excise and VAT, such as "sales taxes". These types of taxes were considered excises if they had a special rate applied on

TAX INCLUSIVE RETAIL SALES PRICE OF CIGARETTES	COUNTRY A (US$)	COUNTRY B (US$)
[A] Manufacturer's price (same in both countries)	2.00	2.00
[B] Country A: ad valorem tax on manufacturer's price (20%) = 20% x [A]	0.40	-
[C] Countries A and B: specific excise	2.00	2.00
[D] Retailer's and wholesaler's profit margin (same in both countries)	0.20	0.20
[E] Country B: ad valorem tax on retailer's price (20%) = 20% x [A]+[C] +[D]	-	0.84
[F] Final price = P = [A]+[B]+[C]+[D]+[E]	4.60	5.04

tobacco products. Sales taxes that applied to all products in the same manner were considered VAT. For example, in the case of Egypt, the general sales tax imposed on consumed products is applied at a much higher rate for tobacco products compared with other products. It therefore acts like an excise tax and in this report is considered as such.

The next step of the exercise was to convert all tax rates into the same base, in our case, the tax inclusive retail sales price (hereafter referred to as P). Consider the example in the table above where Country B applies the same ad valorem tax as Country A, but ends up with higher taxation because the tax is applied later in the distribution chain.

Comparing ad valorem tax rates without taking into account the stage at which the tax is applied could therefore lead to biased results. This is why WHO used the information provided on tax policy in order to calculate the share of tobacco taxes on the most widely sold brand of cigarettes in the country. This indicator takes into account the exact contribution of all taxes in the price of a cigarette pack and therefore represents the best measure of the magnitude of tobacco taxes.

Calculation

S_{ts} is the share of taxes on the price of a widely consumed brand of cigarettes (20-cigarette pack or equivalent).

$$S_{ts} = S_{as} + S_{av} + S_{id} + S_{VAT} \qquad ①$$

Where:

S_{ts} = Total share of taxes on the price of a pack of cigarettes;

S_{as} = Share of amount-specific excise taxes (or equivalent) on the price of a pack of cigarettes;

S_{av} = Share of ad valorem excise taxes (or equivalent) on the price of a pack of cigarettes;

S_{id} = Share of import duties on the price of a pack of cigarettes (if the most popular brand is imported);

S_{VAT} = Share of the value added tax on the price of a pack of cigarettes.

Calculating S_{as} is fairly straightforward and involves dividing the amount for a 20-cigarette pack by the total price. Unlike S_{as}, the share of ad valorem taxes, S_{av} is much more difficult to calculate and involves making some assumptions. On the other hand, S_{id} is sometimes amount-specific, sometimes value-based. It is therefore calculated the same way as S_{as} if it is amount-specific and the same way as S_{av} if it is value-based. S_{VAT} is usually applied at the end of the taxation process, either on the VAT-exclusive or inclusive retail sales price.

To calculate price, it was assumed that the price of a pack of cigarettes could be expressed as the following :

$$P = [(M + M×ID) + (M + M×ID) × T_{av}\% + T_{as} + \pi] × (1 + VAT\%) \qquad ②$$

Where:

P = Price per pack of 20 cigarettes of the most popular brand consumed locally

M = Manufacturer's/distributor's price, or import price if the brand is imported

ID = Total import duties (where applicable) on a pack of 20 cigarettes [1]

T_{av} = Statutory rate of ad valorem tax

T_{as} = Amount specific excise tax on a pack of 20 cigarettes

π = Retailer's, wholesaler's and importer's profit margins (sometimes expressed as a mark-up)

VAT = Statutory rate of value added tax

Changes to this formula were considered based on country-specific conditions such as the base for the ad valorem tax and excise tax, the existence of ad valorem and specific excise taxes, and whether the most popular brand was locally produced or imported. In most of the cases the base for the ad valorem excise tax was the manufacturer's/distributor's price.

Given knowledge of price (P) and amount-specific excise tax (T_{as}) the shares S_{as} (and, where applicable, S_{id}) are easy to recover. The case of ad valorem taxes (and, where applicable, S_{id}) is more complicated because one needs to recover and separate the base ($M + M \times ID$) of the tax into its component parts in order to calculate the amount of ad valorem tax. In most of the cases M was not known (unless specifically reported by the country).

Using equation ②, it is possible to calculate M:

$$M = \frac{\dfrac{P}{1 + VAT\%} - \pi - T_{as}}{(1 + T_{av}\%) \times (1 + ID)} \qquad ③$$

Unfortunately, π is unknown and will systematically vary from country to country. For domestically produced most popular brands, we considered π to be nil (i.e. 0) in the calculation of M because the retailer's and wholesaler's margins are assumed to be negligible. This would result in an overestimation of M and therefore of the base for the ad valorem tax. This will in turn result in an overestimation of the amount of ad valorem tax. Since the goal of this exercise is to measure how high the share of tobacco taxes is in the price of a typical pack of cigarettes, the assumption that the retailer's/wholesaler's profit (π) is nil, therefore, does not penalize countries by underestimating their ad valorem taxes. In light of this it was decided that unless and until country-specific information was made available to WHO, the retailer's/wholesaler's margin would be assumed to be nil for the domestically produced brands.

However, for those countries where the most popular brand is imported, assuming π to be nil would grossly overestimate the base for the ad valorem tax because the importer's profit needs to be taken into account. The import duty is applied on CIF values, and the consequent excise taxes are applied on import duty inclusive CIF values. The importer's profit or own price is added on tax inclusive CIF value. For domestically produced cigarettes, the producer's price includes its own profit so it is automatically included in M but this is not the case for imported products where the tax is imposed on the import duty inclusive CIF value excluding the importer's profit. So calculating M as in equation ③ would mean assuming importer's profit to be zero. The importer's profit is assumed to be relatively significant and ignoring it would therefore overestimate M. For this reason, M had to be estimated differently for imported products: M^* (or the CIF value) was calculated using secondary sources (data from the United Nations Comtrade database). M^* was normally calculated as the import price of cigarettes in a country (value of imports divided by the quantity of imports for the importing country). However, because of limited data availability and because of inconsistencies in the import data in some cases, the export price was also considered. When both values were available, the higher of the two was selected for the CIF value. Looking more closely at the data, import and export prices sometimes varied greatly depending on the partner considered. In order to take this variation into account, the average import and export prices were weighted for each country by the quantities of the imports/exports coming from the different available partners. When the export price was selected, an additional 10 cents was added to the CIF value because the export price does not include cost, insurance and freight price. The 10 cents value was calculated based on the global difference between import and export prices. The ad valorem and other taxes were then calculated in the same manner as for local cigarettes using M^* as the base, where applicable.

In the case of VAT, in most of the cases the base was P excluding the VAT (or, similarly, the manufacturer's/distributor's price plus all excise taxes). In other words:

S_{VAT} = VAT% $\times$ ($P - S_{VAT}$), equivalent to
S_{VAT} = VAT% $\div$ (1+ VAT%)

So in sum the tax rates are calculated this way:

$S_{ts} = S_{id} + S_{as} + S_{av} + S_{VAT}$

$S_{as} = T_{as} \div P$
$S_{av} = (T_{av}\% \times M) \div P$
　　or
　　$(T_{av}\% \times M^* \times (1 + S_{id})) \div P$
　　if the most popular brand was
　　imported
$S_{id} = (T_{ID}\% \times M^*) \div P$
　　(if the import duty is value-based)
　　or
　　$ID \div P$
　　(if it is specific)
S_{VAT} = VAT% $\div$ (1+ VAT%)

[1] Import duties may vary depending on the country of origin in cases of preferential trade agreements. WHO tried to determine the origin of the pack and relevance of using such rates where possible.

APPENDIX I: REGIONAL SUMMARY OF MPOWER MEASURES

Appendix I provides an overview of selected tobacco control policies. For each WHO region an overview table is presented that includes information on monitoring and prevalence, smoke-free environments, treatment of tobacco dependence, health warnings and packaging, advertising, promotion and sponsorship bans, and taxation levels, based on the methodology outlined in Technical Note I.

Country-level data were often but not always provided with supporting documents such as laws, regulations, policy documents, etc. Available documents were reviewed by WHO and questionnaire answers were amended accordingly, especially for Member States that reported meeting the highest standards. This review, however, does not constitute a thorough and complete legal analysis of each country's legislation. Except for smoke-free environments, data were collected at the national/federal level only and, therefore, provide incomplete policy coverage for Member States where subnational governments play an active role in tobacco control.

Age-standardized prevalence estimates for both sexes combined were produced by applying global population weights for males and females to the age-standardized adult male and female daily smoking prevalence rates (as presented in Appendix VII). Global male and female population weights were obtained from the UN population data for 2006.

Africa

Table 1.0.1
Summary of MPOWER measures

... Data not reported/not available.

COUNTRY	ADULT DAILY SMOKING PREVALENCE (2006)	M MONITORING	P SMOKE-FREE POLICIES (LINES REPRESENT LEVEL OF COMPLIANCE)	O CESSATION PROGRAMMES	W HEALTH WARNINGS	E ADVERTISING BANS (LINES REPRESENT LEVEL OF COMPLIANCE)	R TAXATION
Algeria	14%					...	68%
Angola	...					...	37%
Benin	8%		...			...	22%
Botswana	...		...			...	48%
Burkina Faso	14%					‖ »	20%
Burundi	...		...			...	54%
Cameroon	6%					‖‖‖	22%
Cape Verde	8%		‖‖‖‖			‖‖‖‖‖	22%
Central African Republic	...		‖			‖‖‖	28%
Chad	7%					‖‖‖‖	33%
Comoros	16%		‖			‖‖‖	20%
Congo	4%		...		»	‖‖‖‖	32%
Côte d'Ivoire	6%		‖‖‖‖			...	26%
Democratic Republic of the Congo	6%		‖			‖‖‖‖‖	31%
Equatorial Guinea	...		‖			‖‖ »	35%
Eritrea	6%		‖‖‖			‖‖‖‖	55%
Ethiopia	3%		...			...	56%
Gabon	...		...			...	21%
Gambia	15%		‖‖‖			‖‖‖‖	62%
Ghana	4%		...			...	29%
Guinea	...		‖‖	»		‖‖‖	37%
Guinea-Bissau	...		...	»		...	18%
Kenya	11%		‖‖‖			‖‖‖‖	55%
Lesotho	...		‖‖			‖‖‖‖‖‖	38%
Liberia	...		...			...	40%
Madagascar	...		‖‖‖			‖‖‖‖‖‖	67%
Malawi	11%		...			...	51%
Mali	9%		‖			‖‖‖	21%
Mauritania	18%					...	34%
Mauritius	14%		‖‖‖‖‖ ⊙		⊙	‖‖‖‖‖‖	81%
Mozambique	9%		‖‖‖‖			‖‖‖‖	48%
Namibia	13%					...	42%
Niger	...		‖‖‖‖			‖‖‖‖	23%
Nigeria	5%		‖‖‖‖‖			‖‖‖‖‖	32%
Rwanda	...		‖‖‖‖			‖‖‖‖‖	57%
Sao Tome and Principe	15%		...			...	37%
Senegal	8%		...			...	28%
Seychelles	15%		...			...	76%
Sierra Leone	...		...			...	42%
South Africa	16%		‖‖‖‖			‖‖‖‖‖ ⊙	45%
Swaziland	10%		...			...	32%
Togo	...		‖			‖‖‖‖‖‖	30%
Uganda	9%		... ☆			...	63%
United Republic of Tanzania	11%		...			‖	35%
Zambia	10%		‖‖‖			‖‖‖	44%
Zimbabwe	15%		‖‖‖‖			...	43%

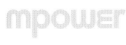

CHANGE SINCE 2007

P SMOKE-FREE POLICIES	O CESSATION PROGRAMMES	W HEALTH WARNINGS	E ADVERTISING BANS	R TAXATION
CHANGE IN POWER INDICATOR GROUP, UP OR DOWN, SINCE 2007				
				▼
				▲
				▼
	▲			
				▲
			▲	
			▲	
				▼
			▲	
				▼
▲		▲		
		▲		
				▼
▲				▼

ADULT DAILY SMOKING PREVALENCE: AGE-STANDARDIZED PREVALENCE RATES FOR ADULT DAILY SMOKERS OF TOBACCO, WEIGHTED BY SEX, 2006

...	Estimate not available
	≥30% or more
	From 20% to 29.9%
	From 15% to 19.9%
	Less than 15%

MONITORING: PREVALENCE DATA

	No known data or no recent data or data that are not both recent and representative
	Recent and representative data for either adults or youth
	Recent and representative data for both adults and youth
	Recent, representative and periodic data for both adults and youth

SMOKE-FREE POLICIES: POLICIES ON SMOKE-FREE ENVIRONMENTS

	Data not reported/not categorized
	Up to two public places completely smoke-free
	Three to five public places completely smoke-free
	Six to seven public places completely smoke-free
	All public places completely smoke-free (or at least 90% of the population covered by complete subnational smoke-free legislation)

CESSATION PROGRAMMES: TREATMENT OF TOBACCO DEPENDENCE

	Data not reported
	None
	Nicotine replacement therapy (NRT) and/or some cessation services (neither cost-covered)
	NRT and/or some cessation services (at least one of which is cost-covered)
	National quit line, and both NRT and some cessation services cost-covered

HEALTH WARNINGS: HEALTH WARNINGS ON CIGARETTE PACKAGES

	Data not reported
	No warning or warning covering <30% of pack surface
	≥30% but no pictures or pictograms and/or other appropriate characteristics
	31–49% including pictures or pictograms and other appropriate characteristics
	≥50% including pictures or pictograms and appropriate characteristics

ADVERTISING BANS: BANS ON ADVERTISING, PROMOTION AND SPONSORSHIP

	Data not reported
	Complete absence of ban, or ban that does not cover national television, radio and print media
	Ban on national television, radio and print media only
	Ban on national television, radio and print media as well as on some but not all other forms of direct and/or indirect advertising
	Ban on all forms of direct and indirect advertising

TAXATION: SHARE OF TOTAL TAXES IN THE RETAIL PRICE OF THE MOST WIDELY SOLD BRAND OF CIGARETTES

	Data not reported
	≤ 25% of retail price is tax
	26–50% of retail price is tax
	51–75% of retail price is tax
	>75% of retail price is tax

COMPLIANCE: COMPLIANCE WITH BANS ON ADVERTISING, PROMOTION AND SPONSORSHIP, AND ADHERENCE TO SMOKE-FREE POLICY

||||||||||	Complete compliance (8/10 to 10/10)
|||||||	Moderate compliance (3/10 to 7/10)
||	Minimal compliance (0/10 to 2/10)
...	Not reported

SYMBOLS LEGEND

☆	Separate, completely enclosed smoking rooms are allowed if they are separately ventilated to the outside and kept under negative air pressure in relation to the surrounding areas. Given the difficulty of meeting the very strict requirements delineated for such rooms, they appear to be a practical impossibility but no reliable empirical evidence is presently available to ascertain whether they have been constructed
⊙	Policy adopted but not implemented by 31 December 2008
»	Data not substantiated by a copy of the legislation
▲ ▼	Change in POWER indicator group, up or down, between 2007 and 2008. Some 2007 data were revised in 2008. 2008 grouping rules were applied to both years

Please refer to Technical Note I for definitions of categories

The Americas

Table 1.0.2
Summary of MPOWER measures

... Data not reported/not available.

COUNTRY	ADULT DAILY SMOKING PREVALENCE (2006)	M MONITORING	P SMOKE-FREE POLICIES (LINES REPRESENT LEVEL OF COMPLIANCE)	O CESSATION PROGRAMMES	W HEALTH WARNINGS	E ADVERTISING BANS (LINES REPRESENT LEVEL OF COMPLIANCE)	R TAXATION
Antigua and Barbuda	...						31%
Argentina	25%						68%
Bahamas	...						25%
Barbados	10%						49%
Belize	4%						35%
Bolivia (Plurinational State of)	29%						41%
Brazil	14%						58%
Canada	15%						65%
Chile	36%						76%
Colombia	...						34%
Costa Rica	6%						56%
Cuba	34%						87%
Dominica	...						49%
Dominican Republic	14%						62%
Ecuador	4%						64%
El Salvador	...						31%
Grenada	...						30%
Guatemala	4%						57%
Guyana	...						27%
Haiti	...						...
Honduras	...						41%
Jamaica	13%						45%
Mexico	14%						65%
Nicaragua	...						23%
Panama	...						44%
Paraguay	16%						19%
Peru	...						43%
Saint Kitts and Nevis	...						30%
Saint Lucia	19%						14%
Saint Vincent and the Grenadines	11%						29%
Suriname	1%						42%
Trinidad and Tobago	...						37%
United States of America	17%						37%
Uruguay	31%						66%
Venezuela (Bolivarian Republic of)	23%						78%

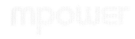

CHANGE SINCE 2007

P SMOKE-FREE POLICIES	O CESSATION PROGRAMMES	W HEALTH WARNINGS	E ADVERTISING BANS	R TAXATION
				▼
▲				
	▲			
▲				
				▼
	▲			
				▼
▲			▲	
			▲	

CHANGE IN POWER INDICATOR GROUP, UP OR DOWN, SINCE 2007

ADULT DAILY SMOKING PREVALENCE: AGE-STANDARDIZED PREVALENCE RATES FOR ADULT DAILY SMOKERS OF TOBACCO, WEIGHTED BY SEX, 2006

. . .	Estimate not available
	≥30% or more
	From 20% to 29.9%
	From 15% to 19.9%
	Less than 15%

MONITORING: PREVALENCE DATA

	No known data or no recent data or data that are not both recent and representative
	Recent and representative data for either adults or youth
	Recent and representative data for both adults and youth
	Recent, representative and periodic data for both adults and youth

SMOKE-FREE POLICIES: POLICIES ON SMOKE-FREE ENVIRONMENTS

	Data not reported/not categorized
	Up to two public places completely smoke-free
	Three to five public places completely smoke-free
	Six to seven public places completely smoke-free
	All public places completely smoke-free (or at least 90% of the population covered by complete subnational smoke-free legislation)

CESSATION PROGRAMMES: TREATMENT OF TOBACCO DEPENDENCE

	Data not reported
	None
	Nicotine replacement therapy (NRT) and/or some cessation services (neither cost-covered)
	NRT and/or some cessation services (at least one of which is cost-covered)
	National quit line, and both NRT and some cessation services cost-covered

HEALTH WARNINGS: HEALTH WARNINGS ON CIGARETTE PACKAGES

	Data not reported
	No warning or warning covering <30% of pack surface
	≥30% but no pictures or pictograms and/or other appropriate characteristics
	31–49% including pictures or pictograms and other appropriate characteristics
	≥50% including pictures or pictograms and appropriate characteristics

---

ADVERTISING BANS: BANS ON ADVERTISING, PROMOTION AND SPONSORSHIP

	Data not reported
	Complete absence of ban, or ban that does not cover national television, radio and print media
	Ban on national television, radio and print media only
	Ban on national television, radio and print media as well as on some but not all other forms of direct and/or indirect advertising
	Ban on all forms of direct and indirect advertising

TAXATION: SHARE OF TOTAL TAXES IN THE RETAIL PRICE OF THE MOST WIDELY SOLD BRAND OF CIGARETTES

	Data not reported
	≤ 25% of retail price is tax
	26–50% of retail price is tax
	51–75% of retail price is tax
	>75% of retail price is tax

COMPLIANCE: COMPLIANCE WITH BANS ON ADVERTISING, PROMOTION AND SPONSORSHIP, AND ADHERENCE TO SMOKE-FREE POLICY

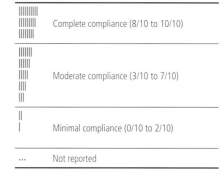

||||||||||	Complete compliance (8/10 to 10/10)
			Moderate compliance (3/10 to 7/10)
	Minimal compliance (0/10 to 2/10)
...	Not reported

SYMBOLS LEGEND

⊙	Policy adopted but not implemented by 31 December 2008
»	Data not substantiated by a copy of the legislation
▲ ▼	Change in POWER indicator group, up or down, between 2007 and 2008. Some 2007 data were revised in 2008. 2008 grouping rules were applied to both years

Please refer to Technical Note I for definitions of categories

South-East Asia

Table 1.0.3
Summary of
MPOWER measures

. . . Data not reported/not available.

COUNTRY	ADULT DAILY SMOKING PREVALENCE (2006)	M MONITORING	P SMOKE-FREE POLICIES LINES REPRESENT LEVEL OF COMPLIANCE	O CESSATION PROGRAMMES	W HEALTH WARNINGS	E ADVERTISING BANS LINES REPRESENT LEVEL OF COMPLIANCE	R TAXATION
Bangladesh	23%		IIIII			IIIIIIIII	67%
Bhutan	. . .		IIIIIIII			IIIIIIIII	. . .
Democratic People's Republic of Korea	. . .		I			IIIIIIII »	. . .
India	15%		IIIII			IIIIII	55%
Indonesia	29%					. . .	53%
Maldives	24%		III »			IIIIIIIIII	30%
Myanmar	23%		III			IIIIIIII	75%
Nepal	28%		IIIII			. . .	25%
Sri Lanka	14%		IIIIIIIII			IIIII	72%
Thailand	18%		IIIIII			IIIIIII	64%
Timor-Leste	. . .						. . .

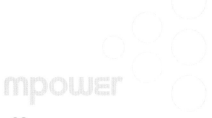

CHANGE SINCE 2007

P SMOKE-FREE POLICIES	O CESSATION PROGRAMMES	W HEALTH WARNINGS	E ADVERTISING BANS	R TAXATION
CHANGE IN POWER INDICATOR GROUP, UP OR DOWN, SINCE 2007				
	▲			
				▼

ADULT DAILY SMOKING PREVALENCE: AGE-STANDARDIZED PREVALENCE RATES FOR ADULT DAILY SMOKERS OF TOBACCO, WEIGHTED BY SEX, 2006

. . .	Estimate not available
	≥30% or more
	From 20% to 29.9%
	From 15% to 19.9%
	Less than 15%

MONITORING: PREVALENCE DATA

	No known data or no recent data or data that are not both recent and representative
	Recent and representative data for either adults or youth
	Recent and representative data for both adults and youth
	Recent, representative and periodic data for both adults and youth

SMOKE-FREE POLICIES:
POLICIES ON SMOKE-FREE ENVIRONMENTS

	Data not reported/not categorized
	Up to two public places completely smoke-free
	Three to five public places completely smoke-free
	Six to seven public places completely smoke-free
	All public places completely smoke-free (or at least 90% of the population covered by complete subnational smoke-free legislation)

CESSATION PROGRAMMES:
TREATMENT OF TOBACCO DEPENDENCE

	Data not reported
	None
	Nicotine replacement therapy (NRT) and/or some cessation services (neither cost-covered)
	NRT and/or some cessation services (at least one of which is cost-covered)
	National quit line, and both NRT and some cessation services cost-covered

HEALTH WARNINGS:
HEALTH WARNINGS ON CIGARETTE PACKAGES

	Data not reported
	No warning or warning covering <30% of pack surface
	≥30% but no pictures or pictograms and/or other appropriate characteristics
	31–49% including pictures or pictograms and other appropriate characteristics
	≥50% including pictures or pictograms and appropriate characteristics

ADVERTISING BANS:
BANS ON ADVERTISING, PROMOTION AND SPONSORSHIP

	Data not reported
	Complete absence of ban, or ban that does not cover national television, radio and print media
	Ban on national television, radio and print media only
	Ban on national television, radio and print media as well as on some but not all other forms of direct and/or indirect advertising
	Ban on all forms of direct and indirect advertising

TAXATION: SHARE OF TOTAL TAXES IN THE RETAIL PRICE OF THE MOST WIDELY SOLD BRAND OF CIGARETTES

	Data not reported
	≤ 25% of retail price is tax
	26–50% of retail price is tax
	51–75% of retail price is tax
	>75% of retail price is tax

COMPLIANCE: COMPLIANCE WITH BANS ON ADVERTISING, PROMOTION AND SPONSORSHIP, AND ADHERENCE TO SMOKE-FREE POLICY

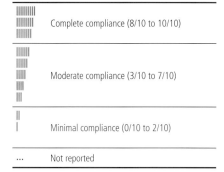

										Complete compliance (8/10 to 10/10)
			Moderate compliance (3/10 to 7/10)
	Minimal compliance (0/10 to 2/10)
…	Not reported

SYMBOLS LEGEND

»	Data not substantiated by a copy of the legislation
▲ ▼	Change in POWER indicator group, up or down, between 2007 and 2008. Some 2007 data were revised in 2008. 2008 grouping rules were applied to both years

Please refer to Technical Note I for definitions of categories

Europe

Table 1.0.4
Summary of MPOWER measures

... Data not reported/not available.

COUNTRY	ADULT DAILY SMOKING PREVALENCE (2006)	M MONITORING	P SMOKE-FREE POLICIES (LINES REPRESENT LEVEL OF COMPLIANCE)	O CESSATION PROGRAMMES	W HEALTH WARNINGS	E ADVERTISING BANS (LINES REPRESENT LEVEL OF COMPLIANCE)	R TAXATION
Albania	21%					||||| »	50%
Andorra	28%		...			...	...
Armenia	29%					|||	32%
Austria	41%						|||||| »	73%
Azerbaijan	...		||			...	22%
Belarus	38%		||||			||||||	23%
Belgium	25%		||||||			|||||	77%
Bosnia and Herzegovina	38%		|||			||||	57%
Bulgaria	37%		||			|||||||	87%
Croatia	30%		|||||| ☆⊙		»	|||||||| »	61%
Cyprus	...		...			...	72%
Czech Republic	25%		||||			|||||	79%
Denmark	26%		...			...	72%
Estonia	29%		|||||			||||||	78%
Finland	21%		||||||||| ☆			|||||||	77%
France	27%		... ☆			...	80%
Georgia	28%		...			|||	55%
Germany	27%		|||||			...	76%
Greece	30%		...			...	73%
Hungary	34%		||||			|||||||	74%
Iceland	20%		|||||||			|||||	71%
Ireland	24%		|||||||||			||||||||	79%
Israel	21%					...	72%
Italy	23%		|||||||| ☆			||||||	75%
Kazakhstan	22%		|||			||||||	20%
Kyrgyzstan	21%		||||			|||||	31%
Latvia	32%					|||||	72%
Lithuania	29%		|||||||			||||||||	71%
Luxembourg	31%		...			...	70%
Malta	23%		|||			|||||||	76%
Monaco	...		...				...
Montenegro	...		|||||			||||||||	44%
Netherlands	25%		...			...	76%
Norway	23%		||||||			|||||||	73%
Poland	29%					|||||||	94%
Portugal	21%		|||||			||||||	77%
Republic of Moldova	21%						||||	22%
Romania	29%		||||			|||||||	74%
Russian Federation	44%		...			...	37%
San Marino	...		...				...
Serbia	29%		||			|||||||	64%
Slovakia	25%		||||||			||||||||	90%
Slovenia	23%		|||||||			|||||||	75%
Spain	28%		|||||			||||||	77%
Sweden	15%		|||||			||||||	73%
Switzerland	22%						62%
Tajikistan	...		|||| »			||||||	...
The former Yugoslav Republic of Macedonia	...		|||||			|||||	39%
Turkey	30%		||||| ⊙			|||||||	73%
Turkmenistan	...		||||			||||||||	43%
Ukraine	39%		...			|||||	45%
United Kingdom of Great Britain and Northern Ireland	18%		|||||||||			|||||||	80%
Uzbekistan	11%		...				32%

mpower

CHANGE SINCE 2007

P SMOKE-FREE POLICIES	O CESSATION PROGRAMMES	W HEALTH WARNINGS	E ADVERTISING BANS	R TAXATION
CHANGE IN POWER INDICATOR GROUP, UP OR DOWN, SINCE 2007				
		▲		
▲				
	▲	▲		▲
				▲
				▲
				▲
				▼
	▲			
			▲	
	▲			
				▲
				▼
	▲			
	▲			
▲				
			▲	
	▲			

ADULT DAILY SMOKING PREVALENCE: AGE-STANDARDIZED PREVALENCE RATES FOR ADULT DAILY SMOKERS OF TOBACCO, WEIGHTED BY SEX, 2006

...	Estimate not available
	≥30% or more
	From 20% to 29.9%
	From 15% to 19.9%
	Less than 15%

MONITORING: PREVALENCE DATA

	No known data or no recent data or data that are not both recent and representative
	Recent and representative data for either adults or youth
	Recent and representative data for both adults and youth
	Recent, representative and periodic data for both adults and youth

SMOKE-FREE POLICIES: POLICIES ON SMOKE-FREE ENVIRONMENTS

	Data not reported/not categorized
	Up to two public places completely smoke-free
	Three to five public places completely smoke-free
	Six to seven public places completely smoke-free
	All public places completely smoke-free (or at least 90% of the population covered by complete subnational smoke-free legislation)

CESSATION PROGRAMMES: TREATMENT OF TOBACCO DEPENDENCE

	Data not reported
	None
	Nicotine replacement therapy (NRT) and/or some cessation services (neither cost-covered)
	NRT and/or some cessation services (at least one of which is cost-covered)
	National quit line, and both NRT and some cessation services cost-covered

HEALTH WARNINGS: HEALTH WARNINGS ON CIGARETTE PACKAGES

	Data not reported
	No warning or warning covering <30% of pack surface
	≥30% but no pictures or pictograms and/or other appropriate characteristics
	31–49% including pictures or pictograms and other appropriate characteristics
	≥50% including pictures or pictograms and appropriate characteristics

ADVERTISING BANS: BANS ON ADVERTISING, PROMOTION AND SPONSORSHIP

	Data not reported
	Complete absence of ban, or ban that does not cover national television, radio and print media
	Ban on national television, radio and print media only
	Ban on national television, radio and print media as well as on some but not all other forms of direct and/or indirect advertising
	Ban on all forms of direct and indirect advertising

TAXATION: SHARE OF TOTAL TAXES IN THE RETAIL PRICE OF THE MOST WIDELY SOLD BRAND OF CIGARETTES

	Data not reported
	≤ 25% of retail price is tax
	26–50% of retail price is tax
	51–75% of retail price is tax
	>75% of retail price is tax

COMPLIANCE: COMPLIANCE WITH BANS ON ADVERTISING, PROMOTION AND SPONSORSHIP, AND ADHERENCE TO SMOKE-FREE POLICY

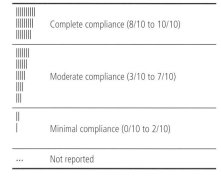

‖‖‖‖‖‖	Complete compliance (8/10 to 10/10)
‖‖‖‖‖	Moderate compliance (3/10 to 7/10)
‖	Minimal compliance (0/10 to 2/10)
...	Not reported

SYMBOLS LEGEND

☆	Separate, completely enclosed smoking rooms are allowed if they are separately ventilated to the outside and kept under negative air pressure in relation to the surrounding areas. Given the difficulty of meeting the very strict requirements delineated for such rooms, they appear to be a practical impossibility but no reliable empirical evidence is presently available to ascertain whether they have been constructed
⊙	Policy adopted but not implemented by 31 December 2008
»	Data not substantiated by a copy of the legislation
▲ ▼	Change in POWER indicator group, up or down, between 2007 and 2008. Some 2007 data were revised in 2008. 2008 grouping rules were applied to both years

Please refer to Technical Note I for definitions of categories

Eastern Mediterranean

Table 1.0.5
Summary of MPOWER measures

... Data not reported/not available.
< Refers to a territory.

2008 INDICATOR AND COMPLIANCE

COUNTRY	ADULT DAILY SMOKING PREVALENCE (2006)	M MONITORING	P SMOKE-FREE POLICIES (lines represent level of compliance)	O CESSATION PROGRAMMES	W HEALTH WARNINGS	E ADVERTISING BANS (lines represent level of compliance)	R TAXATION
Afghanistan	...		II			III	8%
Bahrain	6%		IIIIIIIII			IIIIIIIII	33%
Djibouti	...		III		⊙	IIIIIIIII	44%
Egypt	14%		III			IIIIIIIII	59%
Iran (Islamic Republic of)	14%		IIIIIIIII		⊙	IIIIIIIII	19%
Iraq	11%		I			IIIIII	23%
Jordan	36%		IIII			IIIIII	69%
Kuwait	18%		III			IIIII	34%
Lebanon	17%					...	44%
Libyan Arab Jamahiriya	...		II			...	2%
Morocco	15%		II			IIIIIIIII	66%
Oman	4%		IIIIIIII			...	33%
Pakistan	17%					...	52%
Qatar	...		IIIII		»	IIIIIIIII	33%
Saudi Arabia	7%		... »			... »	33%
Somalia	...		...				...
Sudan	14%		II			IIIIIIIII	72%
Syrian Arab Republic	...		...			IIIIIIIII »	30%
Tunisia	32%				»	IIIIIIII »	65%
United Arab Emirates	8%		...			...	31%
West Bank and Gaza Strip <	...		II		»	... »	...
Yemen	14%		I			IIIII	47%

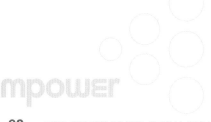

mpower

P SMOKE-FREE POLICIES	O CESSATION PROGRAMMES	W HEALTH WARNINGS	E ADVERTISING BANS	R TAXATION
CHANGE IN POWER INDICATOR GROUP, UP OR DOWN, SINCE 2007				
▲				
▲		▲		▼
		▲		
		▲		
▲				
▲				
	▲			
		▲		
	▲			

ADULT DAILY SMOKING PREVALENCE: AGE-STANDARDIZED PREVALENCE RATES FOR ADULT DAILY SMOKERS OF TOBACCO, WEIGHTED BY SEX, 2006

. . .	Estimate not available
	≥30% or more
	From 20% to 29.9%
	From 15% to 19.9%
	Less than 15%

MONITORING: PREVALENCE DATA

	No known data or no recent data or data that are not both recent and representative
	Recent and representative data for either adults or youth
	Recent and representative data for both adults and youth
	Recent, representative and periodic data for both adults and youth

SMOKE-FREE POLICIES: POLICIES ON SMOKE-FREE ENVIRONMENTS

	Data not reported/not categorized
	Up to two public places completely smoke-free
	Three to five public places completely smoke-free
	Six to seven public places completely smoke-free
	All public places completely smoke-free (or at least 90% of the population covered by complete subnational smoke-free legislation)

CESSATION PROGRAMMES: TREATMENT OF TOBACCO DEPENDENCE

	Data not reported
	None
	Nicotine replacement therapy (NRT) and/or some cessation services (neither cost-covered)
	NRT and/or some cessation services (at least one of which is cost-covered)
	National quit line, and both NRT and some cessation services cost-covered

HEALTH WARNINGS: HEALTH WARNINGS ON CIGARETTE PACKAGES

	Data not reported
	No warning or warning covering <30% of pack surface
	≥30% but no pictures or pictograms and/or other appropriate characteristics
	31–49% including pictures or pictograms and other appropriate characteristics
	≥50% including pictures or pictograms and appropriate characteristics

ADVERTISING BANS: BANS ON ADVERTISING, PROMOTION AND SPONSORSHIP

	Data not reported
	Complete absence of ban, or ban that does not cover national television, radio and print media
	Ban on national television, radio and print media only
	Ban on national television, radio and print media as well as on some but not all other forms of direct and/or indirect advertising
	Ban on all forms of direct and indirect advertising

TAXATION: SHARE OF TOTAL TAXES IN THE RETAIL PRICE OF THE MOST WIDELY SOLD BRAND OF CIGARETTES

	Data not reported
	≤ 25% of retail price is tax
	26–50% of retail price is tax
	51–75% of retail price is tax
	>75% of retail price is tax

COMPLIANCE: COMPLIANCE WITH BANS ON ADVERTISING, PROMOTION AND SPONSORSHIP, AND ADHERENCE TO SMOKE-FREE POLICY

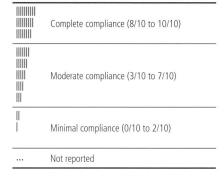

‖‖‖‖‖‖	Complete compliance (8/10 to 10/10)
‖‖‖‖	Moderate compliance (3/10 to 7/10)
‖	Minimal compliance (0/10 to 2/10)
…	Not reported

SYMBOLS LEGEND

⊙	Policy adopted but not implemented by 31 December 2008
≫	Data not substantiated by a copy of the legislation
▲ ▼	Change in POWER indicator group, up or down, between 2007 and 2008. Some 2007 data were revised in 2008. 2008 grouping rules were applied to both years

Please refer to Technical Note I for definitions of categories

2008 INDICATOR AND COMPLIANCE

Table 1.0.6
Summary of MPOWER measures

... Data not reported/not available.

COUNTRY	ADULT DAILY SMOKING PREVALENCE (2006)	M MONITORING	P SMOKE-FREE POLICIES (LINES REPRESENT LEVEL OF COMPLIANCE)	O CESSATION PROGRAMMES	W HEALTH WARNINGS	E ADVERTISING BANS (LINES REPRESENT LEVEL OF COMPLIANCE)	R TAXATION
Australia	18%		...			IIIIIIIII	62%
Brunei Darussalam	...		IIIII			IIIIIIIII	71%
Cambodia	24%		IIIIIIII			...	20%
China	31% [1]		IIIII [1]	[1]	[1]	...	36% [1]
Cook Islands	33%		IIIII			IIIIIIII	65%
Fiji	10%		IIIII			IIIIII	77%
Japan	25%		...			...	63%
Kiribati	...						50%
Lao People's Democratic Republic	35%		IIIIIII			IIIIIII	41%
Malaysia	23%		...			...	48%
Marshall Islands	18%		III			I	40%
Micronesia (Federated States of)	20%		IIIIII			IIIIII	39%
Mongolia	24%		IIIII			IIIII	37%
Nauru	47%		III			IIII	62%
New Zealand	19%		IIIIIIIIII			IIIIIIIII	69%
Niue	...		...			...	66%
Palau	20%		IIIIIIII				57%
Papua New Guinea	...		IIIII	»	»	IIIIIIII »	47%
Philippines	27%		III			IIII	54%
Republic of Korea	28%		IIIII			IIIIII	62%
Samoa	37%		...			...	63%
Singapore	15%		IIIIIIIIII			IIIIIIII	67%
Solomon Islands	...		...			...	...
Tonga	36%		IIIIIII			IIIIIIIII	53%
Tuvalu	34%		IIIII		»	IIIII	...
Vanuatu	26%		IIIII			IIIII	61%
Viet Nam	18%		I			IIIIII	45%

[1] Data not approved by national authorities.

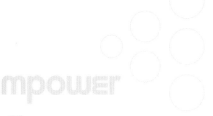

CHANGE SINCE 2007

P SMOKE-FREE POLICIES	O CESSATION PROGRAMMES	W HEALTH WARNINGS	E ADVERTISING BANS	R TAXATION
CHANGE IN POWER INDICATOR GROUP, UP OR DOWN, SINCE 2007				
▲			▲	
		▲		
		▲		
		▲		
			▲	
				▼
	▲			
▲			▲	
	▲			

ADULT DAILY SMOKING PREVALENCE: AGE-STANDARDIZED PREVALENCE RATES FOR ADULT DAILY SMOKERS OF TOBACCO, WEIGHTED BY SEX, 2006

...	Estimate not available
	≥30% or more
	From 20% to 29.9%
	From 15% to 19.9%
	Less than 15%

MONITORING: PREVALENCE DATA

	No known data or no recent data or data that are not both recent and representative
	Recent and representative data for either adults or youth
	Recent and representative data for both adults and youth
	Recent, representative and periodic data for both adults and youth

SMOKE-FREE POLICIES: POLICIES ON SMOKE-FREE ENVIRONMENTS

	Data not reported/not categorized
	Up to two public places completely smoke-free
	Three to five public places completely smoke-free
	Six to seven public places completely smoke-free
	All public places completely smoke-free (or at least 90% of the population covered by complete subnational smoke-free legislation)

CESSATION PROGRAMMES: TREATMENT OF TOBACCO DEPENDENCE

	Data not reported
	None
	Nicotine replacement therapy (NRT) and/or some cessation services (neither cost-covered)
	NRT and/or some cessation services (at least one of which is cost-covered)
	National quit line, and both NRT and some cessation services cost-covered

HEALTH WARNINGS: HEALTH WARNINGS ON CIGARETTE PACKAGES

	Data not reported
	No warning or warning covering <30% of pack surface
	≥30% but no pictures or pictograms and/or other appropriate characteristics
	31–49% including pictures or pictograms and other appropriate characteristics
	≥50% including pictures or pictograms and appropriate characteristics

ADVERTISING BANS: BANS ON ADVERTISING, PROMOTION AND SPONSORSHIP

	Data not reported
	Complete absence of ban, or ban that does not cover national television, radio and print media
	Ban on national television, radio and print media only
	Ban on national television, radio and print media as well as on some but not all other forms of direct and/or indirect advertising
	Ban on all forms of direct and indirect advertising

TAXATION: SHARE OF TOTAL TAXES IN THE RETAIL PRICE OF THE MOST WIDELY SOLD BRAND OF CIGARETTES

	Data not reported
	≤ 25% of retail price is tax
	26–50% of retail price is tax
	51–75% of retail price is tax
	>75% of retail price is tax

COMPLIANCE: COMPLIANCE WITH BANS ON ADVERTISING, PROMOTION AND SPONSORSHIP, AND ADHERENCE TO SMOKE-FREE POLICY

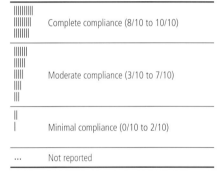

‖‖‖‖‖	Complete compliance (8/10 to 10/10)
‖‖‖‖	Moderate compliance (3/10 to 7/10)
‖	Minimal compliance (0/10 to 2/10)
...	Not reported

SYMBOLS LEGEND

»	Data not substantiated by a copy of the legislation
▲ ▼	Change in POWER indicator group, up or down, between 2007 and 2008. Some 2007 data were revised in 2008. 2008 grouping rules were applied to both years

Please refer to Technical Note I for definitions of categories

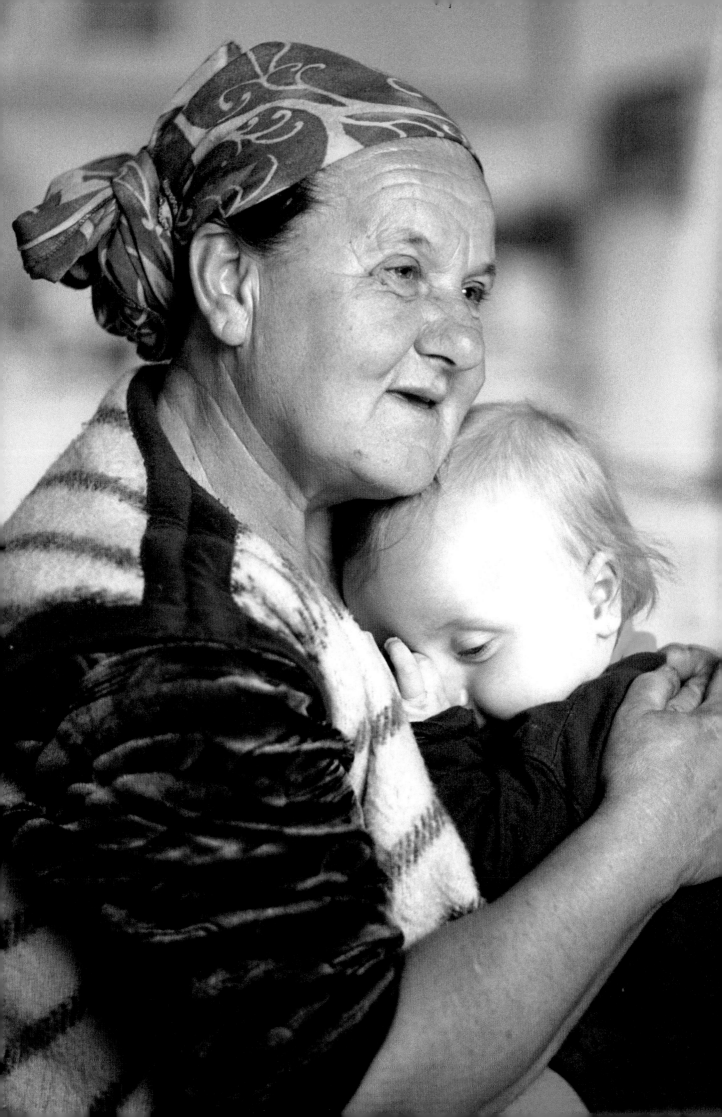

APPENDIX II: **REGULATION OF SMOKE-FREE ENVIRONMENTS**

Appendix II provides detailed information on smoke-free policies, as reported by Member States. Data are provided globally and for each WHO region.

Data on smoke-free environments were often but not always substantiated with supporting documents such as laws, regulations, policy documents, etc. Available documents were reviewed by WHO and implications for questionnaire answers were discussed with countries, especially for Member States that reported meeting the highest standards.

Africa

Table 2.1.1
Public places with smoke-free legislation in Africa

* Based on a score of 0–10, where 0 is low compliance. Refer to Technical Note I for more information.

⊙ Policy adopted but not implemented by 31 December 2008.

☆ Separate, completely enclosed smoking rooms are allowed if they are separately ventilated to the outside and kept under negative air pressure in relation to the surrounding areas. Given the difficulty of meeting the very strict requirements delineated for such rooms, they appear to be a practical impossibility but no reliable empirical evidence is presently available to ascertain whether they have been constructed.

... Data not reported/not available.

— Data not required/not applicable.

COUNTRY	HEALTH-CARE FACILITIES	EDUCATIONAL FACILITIES EXCEPT UNIVERSITIES
Algeria	Yes	Yes
Angola	Yes	No
Benin	Yes	Yes
Botswana	No	No
Burkina Faso	Yes	Yes
Burundi	No	No
Cameroon	Yes	Yes
Cape Verde	No	No
Central African Republic	No	No
Chad	Yes	Yes
Comoros	Yes	Yes
Congo	No	No
Côte d'Ivoire	Yes	Yes
Democratic Republic of the Congo	Yes	Yes
Equatorial Guinea	Yes	Yes
Eritrea	No	No
Ethiopia	No	No
Gabon	No	No
Gambia	No	No
Ghana	No	No
Guinea	Yes	Yes
Guinea-Bissau	No	No
Kenya	No	No
Lesotho	Yes	No
Liberia	No	No
Madagascar	Yes	Yes
Malawi	No	No
Mali	No	No
Mauritania	Yes	No
Mauritius	Yes ⊙	Yes ⊙
Mozambique	No	No
Namibia	No	No
Niger	No	Yes
Nigeria	Yes	Yes
Rwanda	No	No
Sao Tome and Principe	No	No
Senegal	Yes	No
Seychelles	Yes	Yes
Sierra Leone	No	No
South Africa	Yes	Yes
Swaziland	No	No
Togo	No	No
Uganda	Yes	Yes
United Republic of Tanzania	No	No
Zambia	Yes	Yes
Zimbabwe	No	No

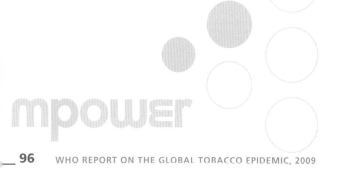

mpower

UNIVERSITIES	GOVERNMENT FACILITIES	INDOOR OFFICES	RESTAURANTS	PUBS AND BARS	PUBLIC TRANSPORT	ALL OTHER INDOOR PUBLIC PLACES	OVERALL COMPLIANCE WITH REGULATIONS ON SMOKE-FREE ENVIRONMENTS *
No	No	No	No	No	No	No	0
No	No	No	No	No	No	No	1
No	Yes	Yes	No	No	No	No	...
No	No	No	No	No	No	No	—
No	Yes	Yes	No	No	No	No	0
No	No	No	No	No	No	No	—
No	No	No	No	No	No	No	0
No	No	No	No	No	Yes	No	5
No	No	No	No	No	No	No	—
Yes	Yes	Yes	Yes	Yes	No	Yes	0
No	No	No	No	No	No	No	2
No	No	No	No	No	No	No	—
No	No	No	No	No	No	No	5
Yes	No	No	No	No	Yes	No	1
Yes	No	No	No	No	No	No	2
No	No	No	No	No	No	No	—
No	No	No	No	No	No	No	—
No	No	No	No	No	No	No	—
No	No	No	No	No	No	No	—
No	No	No	No	No	No	No	—
Yes	Yes	Yes	Yes	Yes	Yes	No	3
No	No	No	No	No	No	No	—
No	No	No	No	No	No	No	—
No	No	No	No	No	No	No	4
No	No	No	No	No	No	No	—
Yes	No	No	No	No	No	No	4
No	No	No	No	No	No	No	—
No	No	No	No	No	No	No	—
No	No	No	No	No	No	No	0
Yes ☉	Yes ☉	Yes ☉	Yes ☉	Yes ☉	Yes ☉	Yes ☉	7
No	No	No	No	No	No	No	—
No	Yes	No	No	No	No	No	...
Yes	No	No	No	No	Yes	No	6
No	Yes	Yes	No	No	Yes	No	7
No	No	No	No	No	No	No	—
No	No	No	No	No	No	No	—
No	No	No	No	No	No	No	0
...	No	No	No	No	No	No	...
No	No	No	No	No	No	No	—
Yes	No	No	No	No	No	No	6
No	No	No	No	No	No	No	—
No	No	No	No	No	No	No	—
Yes	Yes	Yes	☆	☆	☆	☆	...
No	No	No	No	No	No	No	—
Yes	Yes	Yes	Yes	Yes	Yes	Yes	4
No	No	No	No	No	Yes	No	4

The Americas

Table 2.1.2
Public places with smoke-free legislation in the Americas

* Based on a score of 0–10, where 0 is low compliance. Refer to Technical Note I for more information.
⊙ Policy adopted but not implemented by 31 December 2008.
. . . Data not reported/not available.
— Data not required/not applicable.
Please refer to page 124 for country-specific notes.

COUNTRY	HEALTH-CARE FACILITIES	EDUCATIONAL FACILITIES EXCEPT UNIVERSITIES
Antigua and Barbuda	No	No
Argentina	No	No
Bahamas	No	No
Barbados	No	No
Belize	No	No
Bolivia (Plurinational State of)	Yes	Yes
Brazil	No	No
Canada [1]	No	No
Chile	Yes	Yes
Colombia	Yes	Yes
Costa Rica	No	Yes
Cuba	Yes	Yes
Dominica	No	No
Dominican Republic	No	No
Ecuador	Yes	Yes
El Salvador	Yes	No
Grenada	No	No
Guatemala	Yes ⊙	Yes ⊙
Guyana	Yes	Yes
Haiti	No	No
Honduras	Yes	Yes
Jamaica	No	No
Mexico	No	Yes
Nicaragua	Yes	No
Panama	Yes	Yes
Paraguay	Yes	Yes
Peru	Yes	Yes
Saint Kitts and Nevis	No	No
Saint Lucia	No	No
Saint Vincent and the Grenadines	No	No
Suriname	No	No
Trinidad and Tobago	No	No
United States of America	No	No
Uruguay	Yes	Yes
Venezuela (Bolivarian Republic of)	Yes	Yes

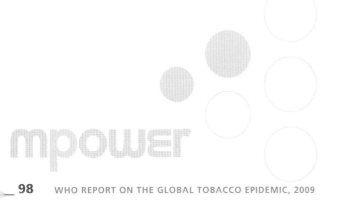

UNIVERSITIES	GOVERNMENT FACILITIES	INDOOR OFFICES	RESTAURANTS	PUBS AND BARS	PUBLIC TRANSPORT	ALL OTHER INDOOR PUBLIC PLACES	OVERALL COMPLIANCE WITH REGULATIONS ON SMOKE-FREE ENVIRONMENTS*
No	No	No	No	No	No	No	—
No	No	No	No	No	No	No	—
No	No	No	No	No	No	No	—
No	No	No	No	No	No	No	—
No	No	No	No	No	No	No	—
Yes	Yes	Yes	Yes	No	Yes	No	...
No	No	No	No	No	Yes	No	9
No	Yes	No	No	No	No	No	...
No	No	No	No	No	No	No	7
Yes	Yes	Yes	Yes	Yes	Yes	Yes	5
No	No	No	No	No	No	No	2
Yes	No	No	No	No	Yes	No	1
No	No	No	No	No	No	No	—
No	No	No	No	No	No	No	—
No	Yes	No	No	No	No	No	5
No	Yes	...	No	No	Yes	No	4
No	No	No	No	No	No	No	—
Yes ⊙	Yes ⊙	Yes ⊙	Yes ⊙	Yes ⊙	Yes ⊙	Yes ⊙	1
No	No	No	No	No	No	No	8
No	No	No	No	No	No	No	—
Yes	Yes	No	No	No	Yes	No	2
No	No	No	No	No	No	No	—
No	No	No	No	No	Yes	No	3
No	No	No	No	No	No	No	3
Yes	Yes	Yes	Yes	Yes	Yes	Yes	10
No	No	No	No	No	No	No	6
Yes	Yes	No	No	No	Yes	No	5
No	No	No	No	No	No	No	—
No	No	No	No	No	No	No	—
No	No	No	No	No	No	No	—
No	No	No	No	No	No	No	—
No	Yes	No	No	No	No	No	6
No	No	No	No	No	No	No	—
Yes	Yes	Yes	Yes	Yes	Yes	Yes	10
No	No	No	No	No	Yes	Yes	6

South-East Asia

Please refer to page 124 for country-specific notes.

Table 2.1.3
Public places with smoke-free legislation in South-East Asia

* Based on a score of 0–10, where 0 is low compliance. Refer to Technical Note I for more information.

» Data not substantiated by a copy of the legislation.

... Data not reported/not available.

— Data not required/not applicable.

Please refer to page 124 for country-specific notes.

COUNTRY	HEALTH-CARE FACILITIES	EDUCATIONAL FACILITIES EXCEPT UNIVERSITIES
Bangladesh	Yes	Yes
Bhutan	Yes	Yes
Democratic People's Republic of Korea	No	No
India	Yes	Yes
Indonesia	Yes	Yes
Maldives	Yes »	Yes »
Myanmar	Yes	Yes
Nepal	No	No
Sri Lanka	Yes	Yes
Thailand	No[2]	Yes
Timor-Leste	No	No

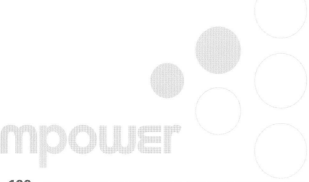

mpower

UNIVERSITIES	GOVERNMENT FACILITIES	INDOOR OFFICES	RESTAURANTS	PUBS AND BARS	PUBLIC TRANSPORT	ALL OTHER INDOOR PUBLIC PLACES	OVERALL COMPLIANCE WITH REGULATIONS ON SMOKE-FREE ENVIRONMENTS *
No	No	No	No	No	No	No	4
Yes	Yes	Yes	Yes	Yes	Yes	Yes	7
No	No	No	No	No	No	No	—
Yes	Yes	Yes	No	No	No	Yes	5
Yes	No	No	No	No	No	No	0
Yes »	Yes »	No	No	...	No	No	3
Yes	No	No	No	No	No	No	3
No	No	No	No	No	No	No	—
Yes	Yes	Yes	No	No	Yes	No	8
No[2]	No[2]	No[2]	No[2]	No[2]	Yes	Yes	6
No	No	No	No	No	No	No	—

Europe

Table 2.1.4
Public places with smoke-free legislation in Europe

* Based on a score of 0–10, where 0 is low compliance. Refer to Technical Note I for more information.

» Data not substantiated by a copy of the legislation.

⊙ Policy adopted but not implemented by 31st December 2008.

☆ Separate, completely enclosed smoking rooms are allowed if they are separately ventilated to the outside and kept under negative air pressure in relation to the surrounding areas. Given the difficulty of meeting the very strict requirements delineated for such rooms, they appear to be a practical impossibility but no reliable empirical evidence is presently available to ascertain whether they have been constructed.

. . . Data not reported/not available.

— Data not required/not applicable.

COUNTRY	HEALTH-CARE FACILITIES	EDUCATIONAL FACILITIES EXCEPT UNIVERSITIES
Albania	No	No
Andorra	Yes	Yes
Armenia	Yes	Yes
Austria	No	No
Azerbaijan	Yes	Yes
Belarus	Yes	No
Belgium	Yes	Yes
Bosnia and Herzegovina	No	No
Bulgaria	No	Yes
Croatia	Yes ⊙	Yes ⊙
Cyprus	No	No
Czech Republic	Yes	Yes
Denmark	Yes	No
Estonia	No	Yes
Finland	Yes	Yes
France	Yes	Yes
Georgia	No	No
Germany	No	No
Greece	No	No
Hungary	No	No
Iceland	No	Yes
Ireland	Yes	Yes
Israel	Yes	No
Italy	☆	☆
Kazakhstan	Yes	Yes
Kyrgyzstan	Yes	Yes
Latvia	No	Yes
Lithuania	No	No
Luxembourg	Yes	Yes
Malta	Yes	Yes
Monaco	. . .	. . .
Montenegro	Yes	Yes
Netherlands	Yes	Yes
Norway	No	No
Poland	No	No
Portugal	Yes	Yes
Republic of Moldova	Yes	Yes
Romania	Yes	No
Russian Federation	No	No
San Marino	. . .	. . .
Serbia	Yes	Yes
Slovakia	Yes	Yes
Slovenia	Yes	Yes
Spain	Yes	Yes
Sweden	Yes	No
Switzerland	No	No
Tajikistan	Yes »	Yes »
The former Yugoslav Republic of Macedonia	No	No
Turkey	Yes	Yes
Turkmenistan	No	Yes
Ukraine	No	No
United Kingdom of Great Britain and Northern Ireland	Yes	Yes
Uzbekistan	No	No

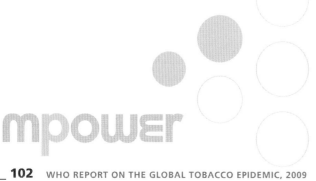

mpower

UNIVERSITIES	GOVERNMENT FACILITIES	INDOOR OFFICES	RESTAURANTS	PUBS AND BARS	PUBLIC TRANSPORT	ALL OTHER INDOOR PUBLIC PLACES	OVERALL COMPLIANCE WITH REGULATIONS ON SMOKE-FREE ENVIRONMENTS *
No	No	No	No	No	No	No	—
...	Yes	No	No	No	...	No	...
Yes	Yes	No	No	No	Yes	Yes	0
Yes	No	No	No	No	No	No	1
No	No	No	No	No	No	No	2
No	No	No	No	No	No	No	4
Yes	Yes	Yes	Yes	No	No	Yes	8
No	No	No	No	No	No	No	—
Yes	No	No	No	No	Yes	Yes	3
☆ ⊙	☆ ⊙	☆ ⊙	☆ ⊙	☆ ⊙	☆ ⊙	☆ ⊙	6
No	No	No	No	No	Yes	No	...
No	Yes	No	No	No	Yes	No	4
No	No	No	No	No	No	No	...
No	No	No	No	No	No	No	8
Yes	Yes	Yes	☆	☆	Yes	Yes	10
☆	☆	☆	☆	☆	☆	☆	...
No	No	No	No	No	No	No	—
No	Yes	Yes	No	No	Yes	No	6
No	No	No	No	No	Yes	No	...
No	No	No	No	No	No	No	—
Yes	No	No	No	No	Yes	No	10
Yes	Yes	Yes	Yes	Yes	Yes	Yes	10
No	No	No	No	No	No	No	8
☆	☆	☆	☆	☆	☆	☆	8
Yes	Yes	No	No	No	No	No	3
Yes	No	No	No	No	No	No	5
No	No	No	No	No	No	No	...
Yes	No	Yes	No	No	No	No	10
No	No	No	No	No	...	No	—
No	No	No	No	No	Yes	No	3
...	...	...	...	...	...	...	...
Yes	Yes	No	No	No	No	No	5
Yes	No	No	No	No	No	No	...
No	No	No	Yes	Yes	No	No	10
No	No	No	No	No	No	No	—
No	Yes	Yes	No	No	Yes	Yes	7
No	No	No	No	No	No	No	1
No	No	No	No	No	Yes	No	5
No	No	No	No	No	No	No	—
...	...	...	...	...	...	...	...
Yes	No	No	No	No	No	No	2
Yes	No	No	No	No	Yes	No	8
Yes	No	No	No	No	No	No	9
Yes	Yes	Yes	No	No	No	Yes	6
No	No	No	No	No	No	No	8
No	No	No	No	No	No	No	—
Yes »	Yes »	Yes »	No	No	Yes	Yes	4
No	No	No	No	No	No	No	—
Yes	Yes	Yes	Yes ⊙	Yes ⊙	Yes	Yes	5
Yes	Yes	Yes	No	No	Yes	No	5
No	No	No	No	No	No	No	—
Yes	Yes	Yes	Yes	Yes	Yes	Yes	10
No	No	No	No	No	No	No	—

Eastern Mediterranean

Table 2.1.5
Public places with smoke-free legislation in the Eastern Mediterranean

* Based on a score of 0–10, where 0 is low compliance. Refer to Technical Note I for more information.

» Data not substantiated by a copy of the legislation.

... Data not reported/not available.

— Data not required/not applicable.

< Refers to a territory.

Please refer to page 124 for country-specific notes.

COUNTRY	HEALTH-CARE FACILITIES	EDUCATIONAL FACILITIES EXCEPT UNIVERSITIES
Afghanistan	Yes	Yes
Bahrain	Yes	Yes
Djibouti	Yes	Yes
Egypt	Yes	Yes
Iran (Islamic Republic of)	Yes	Yes
Iraq	Yes	Yes
Jordan	Yes	Yes
Kuwait	No	No
Lebanon	Yes	Yes
Libyan Arab Jamahiriya	Yes	Yes
Morocco	Yes	No
Oman	Yes	No[3]
Pakistan[4]	Yes	Yes
Qatar	No	No
Saudi Arabia	Yes »	Yes »
Somalia	No	No
Sudan	No	Yes
Syrian Arab Republic	No	No
Tunisia	No	No
United Arab Emirates	Yes	Yes
West Bank and Gaza Strip<	Yes	Yes
Yemen	Yes	Yes

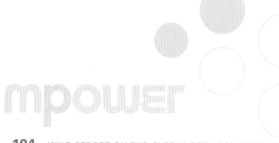

UNIVERSITIES	GOVERNMENT FACILITIES	INDOOR OFFICES	RESTAURANTS	PUBS AND BARS	PUBLIC TRANSPORT	ALL OTHER INDOOR PUBLIC PLACES	OVERALL COMPLIANCE WITH REGULATIONS ON SMOKE-FREE ENVIRONMENTS *
Yes	No	No	No	No	No	No	2
Yes	Yes	Yes	No	No	Yes	Yes	9
Yes	Yes	Yes	Yes	Yes	Yes	No	3
Yes	Yes	Yes	No	No	Yes	Yes	3
Yes	Yes	Yes	Yes	Yes	Yes	Yes	9
No	Yes	No	No	No	No	No	1
Yes	Yes	Yes	No	No	Yes	No	4
No	No	No	No	No	No	Yes	3
Yes	No	No	No	No	Yes	No	0
Yes	Yes	Yes	No	—	Yes	Yes	2
No	No	No	No	No	No	No	1
No	Yes	No	No	No	No	No	8
Yes	No	No	No	—	Yes	No	0
No	No	No	No	No	Yes	Yes	5
Yes »	Yes »	No	No	—	No	No	. . .
. . .	Yes	Yes	No	No	No	No	. . .
No	No	No	No	No	No	Yes	2
No	No	No	No	No	No	No	—
No	No	No	No	No	No	. . .	—
Yes	Yes	Yes	No	No	No	No	. . .
Yes	Yes	Yes	Yes	No	Yes	No	2
Yes	Yes	No	No	No	No	No	1

Western Pacific

Table 2.1.6
Public places with smoke-free legislation in the Western Pacific

COUNTRY	HEALTH-CARE FACILITIES	EDUCATIONAL FACILITIES EXCEPT UNIVERSITIES
Australia[1]	No	No
Brunei Darussalam	Yes	Yes
Cambodia	No	No
China	No[5]	No[5]
Cook Islands	No	No
Fiji	Yes	No
Japan	No	No
Kiribati	No	No
Lao People's Democratic Republic	Yes	Yes
Malaysia	No	No
Marshall Islands	Yes	Yes
Micronesia (Federated States of)	No	No
Mongolia	No	No
Nauru	No	No
New Zealand	Yes	Yes
Niue	No	No
Palau	No	No
Papua New Guinea	No	No
Philippines	Yes	Yes
Republic of Korea	Yes	Yes
Samoa	No	No
Singapore	Yes	Yes
Solomon Islands	No	No
Tonga	No	No
Tuvalu	No	No
Vanuatu	No	No
Viet Nam	Yes	Yes

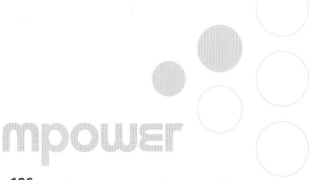

mpower

UNIVERSITIES	GOVERNMENT FACILITIES	INDOOR OFFICES	RESTAURANTS	PUBS AND BARS	PUBLIC TRANSPORT	ALL OTHER INDOOR PUBLIC PLACES	OVERALL COMPLIANCE WITH REGULATIONS ON SMOKE-FREE ENVIRONMENTS *
No	No	No	No	No	No	No	—
Yes	No	Yes	Yes	—	Yes	No	5
No	No	No	No	No	No	No	—
No	No	No	No	No	No[5]	No[5]	—
No	No	No	No	No	Yes	No	5
No	No	No	No	No	No	Yes	5
No	No	No	No	No	No	No	—
No	No	No	No	No	No	No	—
Yes	No	No	No	No	No	No	7
No	No	No	No	No	Yes	No	...
Yes	Yes	Yes	Yes	Yes	Yes	Yes	3
No	No	No	No	No	No	No	—
No	No	No	No	No	No	No	—
No	No	No	No	No	No	No	—
Yes	Yes	Yes	Yes	Yes	Yes	Yes	10
No	No	No	No	No	No	No	—
No	Yes	No	No	No	No	No	7
No	No	No	No	No	No	No	—
Yes	No	No	No	No	No	No	3
No	No	No	No	No	No	No	6
No	No	No	No	No	No	No	—
No	No	No	Yes	No	Yes	No	10
No	No	No	No	No	No	No	—
No	Yes	Yes	No	No	No	Yes	7
No	No	No	Yes	Yes	Yes	No	5
No	No	No	No	No	No	No	—
Yes	Yes	Yes	No	No	Yes	No	1

Africa

Table 2.2.1
Characteristics of smoke-free legislation in Africa

*   At least one province, state or local area has a complete ban on tobacco smoking indoors in health-care, educational or government facilities or workplaces including bars and restaurants.

. . .   Data not reported/not available.

—   Data not required/not applicable.

COUNTRY	NATIONAL BANS
	NUMBER OF PLACES SMOKE-FREE
Algeria	2
Angola	1
Benin	4
Botswana	0
Burkina Faso	4
Burundi	0
Cameroon	2
Cape Verde	1
Central African Republic	0
Chad	7
Comoros	2
Congo	0
Côte d'Ivoire	2
Democratic Republic of the Congo	4
Equatorial Guinea	3
Eritrea	0
Ethiopia	0
Gabon	0
Gambia	0
Ghana	0
Guinea	8
Guinea-Bissau	0
Kenya	0
Lesotho	1
Liberia	0
Madagascar	3
Malawi	0
Mali	0
Mauritania	1
Mauritius	8
Mozambique	0
Namibia	1
Niger	3
Nigeria	5
Rwanda	0
Sao Tome and Principe	0
Senegal	1
Seychelles	2
Sierra Leone	0
South Africa	3
Swaziland	0
Togo	0
Uganda	5
United Republic of Tanzania	0
Zambia	8
Zimbabwe	1

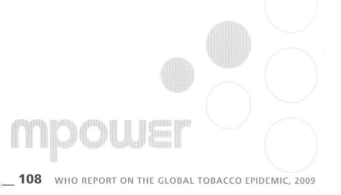

mpower

FINES FOR VIOLATIONS	FINES ON THE ESTABLISHMENT	DEDICATED FUNDS FOR ENFORCEMENT	CITIZEN COMPLAINTS AND INVESTIGATIONS	SUBNATIONAL BANS	
				AUTHORITY EXISTS	COMPREHENSIVE BANS IN PLACE*
No	—	No	No	Yes	No
No	—	No	No	Yes	No
Yes	No	No	Yes	No	—
Yes	...	...	...	...	...
Yes	No	No	No	No	—
No	—	No	No	No	—
No	—	No	No	Yes	No
Yes	Yes	No	No	No	—
Yes	No	No	No	Yes	Yes
No	—	No	No	No	—
Yes	No	No	No	Yes	No
No	—	Yes	No	No	—
No	—	Yes	Yes	No	—
Yes	No	No	No	Yes	No
No	—	No	Yes	Yes	No
Yes	Yes	No	No	No	—
No	—	No	No	No	—
No	—	No	No	No	—
Yes	No	No	No	Yes	No
No	—	No	No	No	—
No	—	No	No	No	—
No	—	No	No	Yes	No
Yes	No	Yes	No	Yes	No
Yes	No	No	No	No	—
No	—	No	No	No	—
No	—	No	No	No	—
No	—	No	No	No	—
Yes	Yes	Yes	No	No	—
No	—	No	No	No	—
Yes	Yes	No	Yes	No	—
No	—	No	No	No	—
No	—	No	No	Yes	No
Yes	Yes	No	Yes	No	—
Yes	No	No	No	Yes	No
No	—	No	No	No	—
No	—	No	No	No	—
Yes	No	No	No	No	—
No	—	No	No	No	—
No	—	No	No	No	—
Yes	Yes	Yes	Yes	No	—
No	—	No	No	No	—
No	—	No	No	No	—
Yes	Yes	No	No	Yes	No
Yes	Yes	No	No	Yes	No
Yes	Yes	No	Yes	Yes	No
Yes	Yes	Yes	Yes	Yes	No

The Americas

Table 2.2.2
Characteristics of smoke-free legislation in the Americas

* At least one province, state or local area has a complete ban on tobacco smoking indoors in health-care, educational or government facilities or workplaces including bars and restaurants.

... Data not reported/not available.

— Data not required/not applicable.

COUNTRY	NATIONAL BANS
	NUMBER OF PLACES SMOKE-FREE
Antigua and Barbuda	0
Argentina	0
Bahamas	0
Barbados	0
Belize	0
Bolivia (Plurinational State of)	7
Brazil	1
Canada	1
Chile	2
Colombia	8
Costa Rica	1
Cuba	4
Dominica	0
Dominican Republic	0
Ecuador	3
El Salvador	3
Grenada	0
Guatemala	8
Guyana	2
Haiti	0
Honduras	5
Jamaica	0
Mexico	2
Nicaragua	1
Panama	8
Paraguay	2
Peru	5
Saint Kitts and Nevis	0
Saint Lucia	0
Saint Vincent and the Grenadines	0
Suriname	0
Trinidad and Tobago	1
United States of America	0
Uruguay	8
Venezuela (Bolivarian Republic of)	3

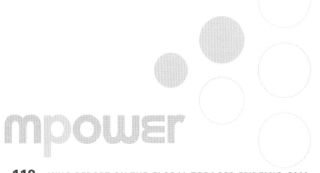
mpower

FINES FOR VIOLATIONS	FINES ON THE ESTABLISHMENT	DEDICATED FUNDS FOR ENFORCEMENT	CITIZEN COMPLAINTS AND INVESTIGATIONS	SUBNATIONAL BANS	
				AUTHORITY EXISTS	COMPREHENSIVE BANS IN PLACE*
No	—	No	No	No	—
No	—	No	No	Yes	Yes
No	—	No	No	No	—
No	—	No	No	No	—
No	—	No	No	No	—
Yes	Yes	No	No	No	—
Yes	Yes	No	Yes	Yes	No
Yes	Yes	Yes	Yes	Yes	Yes
Yes	Yes	No	Yes	No	—
Yes	Yes	No	No	Yes	No
Yes	Yes	No	Yes	No	—
Yes	Yes	No	Yes	No	—
No	—	No	No	No	—
Yes	Yes	No	No	No	—
Yes	No	No	No	No	—
No	—	No	No	No	—
No	—	No	No	No	—
Yes	Yes	Yes	No	No	—
No	—	No	No	No	—
...	...	...	...	...	...
No	—	No	No	No	—
No	—	No	No	No	—
Yes	Yes	Yes	Yes	Yes	Yes
No	—	No	No	No	—
Yes	Yes	Yes	Yes	No	—
No	—	No	Yes	No	—
Yes	Yes	No	No	No	—
No	—	No	No	No	—
No	—	No	No	No	—
No	—	No	No	No	—
No	—	No	No	No	—
No	—	No	No	No	—
No	—	No	No	Yes	Yes
Yes	Yes	Yes	Yes	No	—
Yes	Yes	Yes	Yes	Yes	Yes

South-East Asia

Table 2.2.3
Characteristics of smoke-free legislation in South-East Asia

* At least one province, state or local area has a complete ban on tobacco smoking indoors in health-care, educational or government facilities or workplaces including bars and restaurants.

— Data not required/not applicable.

COUNTRY	NATIONAL BANS
	NUMBER OF PLACES SMOKE-FREE
Bangladesh	2
Bhutan	8
Democratic People's Republic of Korea	0
India	5
Indonesia	3
Maldives	4
Myanmar	3
Nepal	0
Sri Lanka	6
Thailand	2
Timor-Leste	0

mpower

FINES FOR VIOLATIONS	FINES ON THE ESTABLISHMENT	DEDICATED FUNDS FOR ENFORCEMENT	CITIZEN COMPLAINTS AND INVESTIGATIONS	SUBNATIONAL BANS	
				AUTHORITY EXISTS	COMPREHENSIVE BANS IN PLACE*
Yes	No	No	No	No	—
No	—	No	No	No	—
Yes	Yes	No	Yes	Yes	No
Yes	Yes	No	Yes	No	—
No	—	No	No	Yes	No
No	—	No	No	No	—
Yes	No	No	No	No	—
No	—	No	No	No	—
Yes	Yes	Yes	No	No	—
Yes	Yes	No	Yes	Yes	No
No	—	No	No	No	—

Europe

Table 2.2.4
Characteristics of smoke-free legislation in Europe

*   At least one province, state or local area has a complete ban on tobacco smoking indoors in health-care, educational or government facilities or workplaces including bars and restaurants.

...   Data not reported/not available.

—   Data not required/not applicable.

COUNTRY	NATIONAL BANS
	NUMBER OF PLACES SMOKE-FREE
Albania	0
Andorra	3
Armenia	5
Austria	1
Azerbaijan	2
Belarus	1
Belgium	6
Bosnia and Herzegovina	0
Bulgaria	3
Croatia	2
Cyprus	1
Czech Republic	4
Denmark	1
Estonia	1
Finland	6
France	2
Georgia	0
Germany	3
Greece	1
Hungary	0
Iceland	3
Ireland	8
Israel	1
Italy	0
Kazakhstan	4
Kyrgyzstan	3
Latvia	1
Lithuania	2
Luxembourg	2
Malta	3
Monaco	0
Montenegro	4
Netherlands	3
Norway	2
Poland	0
Portugal	5
Republic of Moldova	2
Romania	2
Russian Federation	0
San Marino	0
Serbia	3
Slovakia	4
Slovenia	3
Spain	5
Sweden	1
Switzerland	0
Tajikistan	6
The former Yugoslav Republic of Macedonia	0
Turkey	8
Turkmenistan	5
Ukraine	0
United Kingdom of Great Britain and Northern Ireland	8
Uzbekistan	0

mpower

FINES FOR VIOLATIONS	FINES ON THE ESTABLISHMENT	DEDICATED FUNDS FOR ENFORCEMENT	CITIZEN COMPLAINTS AND INVESTIGATIONS	SUBNATIONAL BANS	
				AUTHORITY EXISTS	COMPREHENSIVE BANS IN PLACE*
Yes	Yes	No	Yes	No	—
...	...	...	...	...	...
No	—	No	No	No	—
Yes	Yes	No	Yes	Yes	No
Yes	No	No	Yes	No	—
Yes	No	No	Yes	Yes	No
Yes	Yes	No	Yes	Yes	No
No	—	No	No	No	—
Yes	Yes	Yes	Yes	Yes	No
Yes	Yes	Yes	Yes	No	—
Yes	Yes	No	No	No	—
No	—	No	Yes	No	—
Yes	Yes	No	Yes	Yes	No
Yes	Yes	No	Yes	Yes	No
Yes	Yes	Yes	Yes	No	—
Yes	Yes	No	No	No	—
No	—	No	No	No	—
Yes	No	No	No	Yes	No
Yes	No	No	Yes	No	—
Yes	Yes	No	Yes	No	—
Yes	No	Yes	Yes	No	—
Yes	Yes	No	Yes	No	—
Yes	Yes	No	Yes	Yes	No
Yes	Yes	No	Yes	No	—
Yes	Yes	Yes	Yes	No	—
Yes	Yes	Yes	No	Yes	No
Yes	Yes	No	Yes	Yes	No
Yes	Yes	No	Yes	No	—
...	...	...	...	...	...
Yes	Yes	No	Yes	No	—
...	...	...	...	...	...
Yes	Yes	No	Yes	No	—
Yes	Yes	Yes	Yes	No	—
Yes	Yes	No	No	No	—
Yes	Yes	Yes	Yes	Yes	No
Yes	Yes	No	Yes	No	—
No	—	No	No	No	—
Yes	Yes	No	Yes	No	—
Yes	Yes	No	No	No	—
...	...	...	...	...	...
Yes	Yes	No	No	No	—
No	—	Yes	Yes	Yes	No
Yes	Yes	Yes	Yes	No	—
Yes	Yes	No	Yes	Yes	No
Yes	Yes	No	Yes	No	—
No	—	No	No	Yes	Yes
Yes	Yes	No	Yes	Yes	No
No	—	No	Yes	No	—
Yes	Yes	No	No	Yes	No
Yes	No	Yes	Yes	Yes	No
Yes	No	No	No	Yes	No
No	—	No	No	Yes	Yes
No	—	No	No	No	—

Eastern Mediterranean

Table 2.2.5
Characteristics of smoke-free legislation in the Eastern Mediterranean

* At least one province, state or local area has a complete ban on tobacco smoking indoors in health-care, educational or government facilities or workplaces including bars and restaurants.

... Data not reported/not available.

— Data not required/not applicable.

< Refers to a territory.

COUNTRY	NATIONAL BANS
	NUMBER OF PLACES SMOKE-FREE
Afghanistan	3
Bahrain	6
Djibouti	8
Egypt	6
Iran (Islamic Republic of)	8
Iraq	3
Jordan	6
Kuwait	0
Lebanon	4
Libyan Arab Jamahiriya	6
Morocco	1
Oman	2
Pakistan	4
Qatar	1
Saudi Arabia	4
Somalia	2
Sudan	1
Syrian Arab Republic	0
Tunisia	0
United Arab Emirates	5
West Bank and Gaza Strip <	7
Yemen	4

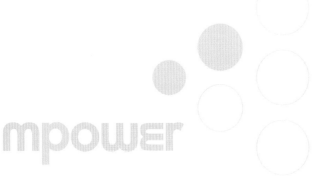

FINES FOR VIOLATIONS	FINES ON THE ESTABLISHMENT	DEDICATED FUNDS FOR ENFORCEMENT	CITIZEN COMPLAINTS AND INVESTIGATIONS	SUBNATIONAL BANS	
				AUTHORITY EXISTS	COMPREHENSIVE BANS IN PLACE *
No	—	No	No	No	—
Yes	Yes	No	No	No	—
No	—	No	No	No	—
Yes	Yes	Yes	No	No	—
Yes	Yes	Yes	Yes	No	—
Yes	No	No	Yes	Yes	Yes
Yes	No	No	No	No	—
Yes	No	No	No	No	—
No	—	No	No	No	—
No	—	No	No	No	—
Yes	No	No	No	No	—
No	—	No	No	No	—
Yes	No	Yes	Yes	No	—
Yes	Yes	No	No	Yes	No
No	—	No	No	Yes	No
...	...	...	...	...	...
Yes	Yes	No	No	Yes	No
No	—	No	No	No	—
Yes	No	No	Yes	No	—
Yes	No	Yes	Yes	Yes	Yes
Yes	Yes	No	No	No	—
Yes	Yes	Yes	No	Yes	No

Western Pacific

Table 2.2.6
Characteristics of smoke-free legislation in the Western Pacific

* At least one province, state or local area has a complete ban on tobacco smoking indoors in health-care, educational or government facilities or workplaces including bars and restaurants.

» Data not substantiated by a copy of the legislation.

— Data not required/not applicable.

COUNTRY	NATIONAL BANS
	NUMBER OF PLACES SMOKE-FREE
Australia	0
Brunei Darussalam	6
Cambodia	0
China	0
Cook Islands	1
Fiji	1
Japan	0
Kiribati	0
Lao People's Democratic Republic	3
Malaysia	1
Marshall Islands	8
Micronesia (Federated States of)	0
Mongolia	0
Nauru	0
New Zealand	8
Niue	0
Palau	1
Papua New Guinea	0
Philippines	3
Republic of Korea	2
Samoa	0
Singapore	4
Solomon Islands	0
Tonga	2
Tuvalu	3
Vanuatu	0
Viet Nam	6

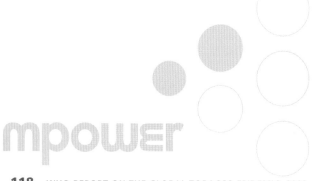

FINES FOR VIOLATIONS	FINES ON THE ESTABLISHMENT	DEDICATED FUNDS FOR ENFORCEMENT	CITIZEN COMPLAINTS AND INVESTIGATIONS	SUBNATIONAL BANS	
				AUTHORITY EXISTS	COMPREHENSIVE BANS IN PLACE*
No	—	No	No	Yes	Yes
Yes	Yes	No	Yes	No	—
No	—	No	No	No	—
Yes	Yes	Yes	Yes	Yes	Yes
Yes	Yes	Yes	No	No	—
Yes	Yes	No	Yes	Yes	No
No	—	No	No	Yes	No
No	—	No	No	No	—
Yes	Yes	Yes	Yes	No	—
Yes	Yes	No	Yes	Yes	No
Yes	Yes	Yes	Yes	Yes	No
Yes	Yes	No	No	Yes	No
Yes	Yes	Yes	Yes	No	—
No	—	No	No	No	—
Yes	Yes	No	Yes	Yes	No
No	—	No	No	No	—
No	—	No	No	No	—
Yes »	Yes »	No	No	Yes »	No
Yes	Yes	Yes	Yes	Yes	No
No	—	No	No	No	—
No	—	No	No	No	—
Yes	Yes	Yes	Yes	No	—
No	—	No	No	No	—
Yes	Yes	No	No	No	—
Yes	Yes	No	Yes	Yes	No
No	—	No	No	No	—
Yes	No	No	No	No	—

Table 2.3.0
Subnational smoke-free environments

Please refer to page 124 for country-specific notes.

COUNTRY	JURISDICTION
Argentina	Córdoba
	Entre Ríos
	Mendoza
	Neuquén
	Santa Fé
	Tucumán
Australia	Australian Capital Territory
	New South Wales
	Northern Territory
	Queensland
	South Australia
	Tasmania
	Victoria
	Western Australia
Belgium	Flemish Region
Brazil	Rio de Janeiro
Canada	Alberta
	British Columbia
	Manitoba
	New Brunswick
	Newfoundland and Labrador
	Northwest Territories
	Nova Scotia
	Nunavut
	Ontario
	Prince Edward Island
	Quebec
	Saskatchewan
	Yukon
Central African Republic	Bangui
China	Beijing
	Hong Kong Special Administrative Region
Comoros	Autonomous Island of Ngazidja
Germany	Baden-Württemberg
	Bavaria
	Berlin
	Brandenburg
	Bremen
	Hamburg
	Hesse
	Lower Saxony
	Mecklenburg-Vorpommern
	North Rhine-Westphalia
	Rhineland-Palatinate
	Saarland
	Saxony
	Saxony-Anhalt
	Schleswig-Holstein
	Thuringia

mpower

HEALTH-CARE FACILITIES	EDUCATIONAL FACILITIES, EXCEPT UNIVERSITIES	UNIVERSITIES	GOVERNMENT FACILITIES	INDOOR OFFICES	RESTAURANTS	PUBS AND BARS	PUBLIC TRANSPORT	OTHER INDOOR WORKPLACES
Yes	Yes	Yes	Yes	Yes	Yes	No	Yes	No
Yes	Yes	Yes	Yes	No	Yes	No	Yes	No
No	Yes	Yes	Yes	No	Yes	No	Yes	No
Yes	Yes	Yes	Yes	Yes	Yes	Yes	Yes	Yes
Yes	Yes	Yes	Yes	Yes	Yes	Yes	Yes	Yes
Yes	Yes	Yes	Yes	Yes	Yes	Yes	Yes	Yes
Yes	Yes	Yes	Yes	Yes	Yes	Yes	Yes	Yes
Yes	Yes	Yes	Yes	Yes	Yes	Yes	Yes	Yes
Yes	Yes	No	Yes	Yes	Yes	No	Yes	Yes
Yes	Yes	Yes	Yes	Yes	Yes	Yes	Yes	Yes
Yes	Yes	Yes	Yes	Yes	Yes	Yes	Yes	Yes
Yes	Yes	Yes	Yes	Yes	Yes	No	Yes	Yes
Yes	Yes	Yes	Yes	Yes	Yes	Yes	Yes	Yes
Yes	Yes	Yes	Yes	Yes	Yes	Yes	Yes	Yes
No	Yes	No	No	No	No	No	No	No
Yes	Yes	Yes	Yes	Yes	Yes	No	No	Yes
Yes	Yes	Yes	Yes	Yes	Yes	Yes	Yes	Yes
Yes	Yes	Yes	Yes	Yes	Yes	Yes	Yes	Yes
Yes	Yes	Yes	Yes	Yes	Yes	Yes	Yes	Yes
Yes	Yes	Yes	Yes	Yes	Yes	Yes	Yes	Yes
Yes	Yes	Yes	Yes	No	Yes	Yes	Yes	No
Yes	Yes	Yes	Yes	No	Yes	Yes	Yes	Yes
Yes	Yes	Yes	Yes	Yes	Yes	Yes	Yes	Yes
Yes	Yes	Yes	Yes	No	Yes	Yes	Yes	No
Yes	Yes	Yes	Yes	Yes	Yes	Yes	Yes	Yes
Yes	Yes	Yes	Yes	No	Yes	Yes	Yes	Yes
Yes	Yes	Yes	Yes	Yes	Yes	Yes	Yes	Yes
Yes	Yes	Yes	Yes	Yes	Yes	Yes	Yes	No
Yes	Yes	Yes	Yes	Yes	Yes	Yes	Yes	Yes
Yes	Yes	Yes	Yes	Yes	Yes	Yes	Yes	Yes
Yes	Yes	No	Yes	Yes	No	No	Yes	No
Yes[5]	Yes[5]	Yes	Yes	Yes	Yes	Yes	Yes[5]	Yes[5]
Yes	Yes	No	Yes	Yes	No	No	No	No
No	No	Yes	No	No	No	No	Yes	No
No	Yes	No	No	No	Yes	Yes	Yes	No
Yes	Yes	Yes	Yes	Yes	No	No	Yes	No
Yes	Yes	Yes	Yes	Yes	No	No	Yes	No
No	Yes	Yes	Yes	Yes	No	No	Yes	No
No	Yes	No	No	No	No	No	Yes	No
No	Yes	Yes	No	Yes	No	No	Yes	No
No	Yes	No	No	Yes	No	No	Yes	No
No	Yes	No	No	Yes	No	No	Yes	No
No	No	No	No	Yes	No	No	Yes	No
Yes	No	Yes	Yes	Yes	No	No	Yes	No
No	Yes	Yes	No	Yes	No	No	Yes	No
No	Yes	Yes	Yes	No	No	No	Yes	No
Yes	Yes	Yes	Yes	Yes	No	No	Yes	No
No	Yes	No	No	Yes	No	No	Yes	No
Yes	Yes	Yes	No	Yes	No	No	Yes	No

Table 2.3.0
Subnational smoke-free environments

COUNTRY	JURISDICTION
Indonesia	Jakarta
Iraq	Al Anbar
	Al Basrah
	Al Muthanna
	Al-Qadisiyyah
	Arbil
	As Sulaymaniyah
	Babil
	Baghdad
	Dhi Qar
	Diyala
	Duhok
	Karbala
	Kirkuk
	Maysan
	Najaf
	Ninawa
	Salah ad Din
	Wasit
Mexico	Federal District (Mexico City)
	Veracruz
Nigeria	Cross River State
	Federal Capital Territory
Switzerland	Ticino
Ukraine	Kiev
	Lutsk
United Arab Emirates	Abu Dhabi
	Sharjah
United Kingdom of Great Britain and Northern Ireland	England
	Northern Ireland
	Scotland
	Wales
United States of America	Alaska
	Arizona
	Arkansas
	California
	Colorado
	Connecticut
	Delaware
	District of Columbia
	Florida
	Georgia
	Hawaii
	Idaho
	Illinois
	Iowa
	Kansas
	Louisiana

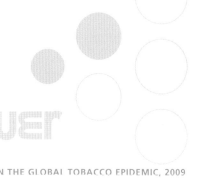

HEALTH-CARE FACILITIES	EDUCATIONAL FACILITIES, EXCEPT UNIVERSITIES	UNIVERSITIES	GOVERNMENT FACILITIES	INDOOR OFFICES	RESTAURANTS	PUBS AND BARS	PUBLIC TRANSPORT	OTHER INDOOR WORKPLACES
Yes	Yes	Yes	No	No	No	No	No	No
Yes	Yes	No	No	No	No	No	No	No
Yes	Yes	No	No	No	No	No	No	No
Yes	Yes	No	No	No	No	No	No	No
Yes	Yes	No	No	No	No	No	No	No
Yes	Yes	Yes	Yes	Yes	Yes	Yes	Yes	No
Yes	Yes	Yes	Yes	Yes	Yes	Yes	Yes	No
Yes	Yes	No	No	No	No	No	No	No
Yes	Yes	No	No	No	No	No	No	No
Yes	Yes	No	No	No	No	No	No	No
Yes	Yes	No	No	No	No	No	No	No
Yes	Yes	Yes	Yes	Yes	Yes	Yes	Yes	No
Yes	Yes	No	No	No	No	No	No	No
Yes	Yes	No	No	No	No	No	No	No
Yes	Yes	No	No	No	No	No	No	No
Yes	Yes	No	No	No	No	No	No	No
Yes	Yes	No	No	No	No	No	No	No
Yes	Yes	No	No	No	No	No	No	No
Yes	Yes	Yes	Yes	Yes	Yes	Yes	Yes	Yes
Yes	No	No	Yes	No	No	No	Yes	Yes
Yes	Yes	No	Yes	Yes	No	No	Yes	No
Yes	Yes	No	Yes	Yes	No	No	Yes	No
Yes	Yes	Yes	Yes	Yes	Yes	Yes	Yes	Yes
Yes	Yes	Yes	No	No	No	No	No	Yes
No	No	No	No	No	No	No	No	Yes
Yes	Yes	Yes	Yes	Yes	Yes	Yes	Yes	Yes
Yes	Yes	Yes	No	Yes	Yes	Yes	Yes	Yes
Yes	Yes	Yes	Yes	Yes	Yes	Yes	Yes	Yes
Yes	Yes	Yes	Yes	Yes	Yes	Yes	Yes	Yes
Yes	Yes	Yes	Yes	Yes	Yes	Yes	Yes	Yes
Yes	Yes	Yes	Yes	Yes	Yes	Yes	Yes	Yes
Yes	No	No	No	No	No	No	No	No
Yes	Yes	No	Yes	Yes	Yes	Yes	Yes	Yes
Yes	Yes	Yes	Yes	Yes	Yes	Yes	Yes	Yes
No	Yes	No	No	Yes	No	No	No	No
Yes	Yes	No	Yes	Yes	Yes	Yes	Yes	Yes
Yes	Yes	Yes	No	No	No	No	No	No
Yes	Yes	Yes	Yes	Yes	Yes	Yes	Yes	Yes
Yes	Yes	Yes	Yes	Yes	Yes	Yes	Yes	Yes
No	Yes	No	Yes	Yes	Yes	No	Yes	No
No	Yes	Yes	No	No	No	No	Yes	No
Yes	Yes	Yes	Yes	Yes	Yes	Yes	Yes	Yes
Yes	Yes	Yes	Yes	No	Yes	No	Yes	Yes
Yes	Yes	Yes	Yes	Yes	Yes	Yes	Yes	Yes
Yes	Yes	Yes	Yes	Yes	Yes	Yes	Yes	No
No	Yes	No	No	No	No	No	Yes	No
No	Yes	No	Yes	Yes	Yes	No	Yes	Yes

Table 2.3.0
Subnational smoke-free environments

COUNTRY	JURISDICTION
United States of America (contd.)	Maine
	Maryland
	Massachusetts
	Michigan
	Minnesota
	Mississippi
	Missouri
	Montana
	Nebraska
	Nevada
	New Hampshire
	New Jersey
	New Mexico
	New York
	North Carolina
	North Dakota
	Ohio
	Oklahoma
	Oregon
	Pennsylvania
	Rhode Island
	South Dakota
	Tennessee
	Utah
	Vermont
	Virginia
	Washington
	West Virginia
	Wisconsin
Venezuela (Bolivarian Republic of)	Monagas

NOTES TO APPENDIX II

[1] Smoke-free legislation does not meet criteria for a complete ban, which is defined such that smoking is not allowed at any time in any indoor area under any circumstances. However, there is very strong subnational smoke-free legislation meeting these conditions.

[2] Air-conditioned public places are completely smoke-free.

[3] Designated smoking rooms are allowed without specific technical requirements but are practically all located outside the buildings.

[4] On 31 May 2009, the federal Minister for Health formally withdrew the Statutory Regulatory Order from September 2008 which permitted designated smoking areas in public places.

[5] Data not approved by national authorities.

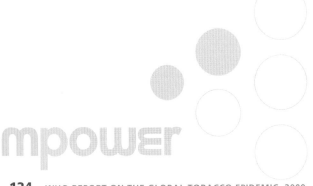

HEALTH-CARE FACILITIES	EDUCATIONAL FACILITIES, EXCEPT UNIVERSITIES	UNIVERSITIES	GOVERNMENT FACILITIES	INDOOR OFFICES	RESTAURANTS	PUBS AND BARS	PUBLIC TRANSPORT	OTHER INDOOR WORKPLACES
No	Yes	No	No	No	Yes	Yes	No	No
Yes	Yes	Yes	Yes	Yes	Yes	Yes	Yes	Yes
Yes	Yes	Yes	Yes	Yes	Yes	Yes	Yes	Yes
No	Yes	No	Yes	No	No	No	No	No
Yes	Yes	Yes	Yes	Yes	Yes	Yes	Yes	Yes
No	Yes	Yes	Yes	No	No	No	Yes	No
No	Yes	No	No	No	No	No	No	No
Yes	Yes	Yes	Yes	Yes	Yes	No	Yes	Yes
Yes	Yes	Yes	Yes	Yes	Yes	Yes	Yes	Yes
Yes	Yes	Yes	Yes	Yes	Yes	No	Yes	Yes
Yes	Yes	No	No	No	Yes	No	Yes	No
Yes	Yes	No	Yes	Yes	Yes	Yes	Yes	No
Yes	Yes	Yes	Yes	Yes	Yes	Yes	Yes	No
Yes	Yes	Yes	Yes	Yes	Yes	Yes	Yes	Yes
No	Yes	No	Yes	No	No	No	No	No
Yes	Yes	No	Yes	Yes	No	No	Yes	No
Yes	Yes	Yes	Yes	Yes	Yes	Yes	Yes	Yes
No	Yes	No	No	No	No	No	Yes	Yes
Yes	Yes	Yes	Yes	Yes	Yes	Yes	Yes	Yes
Yes	Yes	Yes	Yes	Yes	No	No	Yes	No
Yes	Yes	Yes	Yes	Yes	Yes	Yes	Yes	No
Yes	Yes	No	Yes	Yes	Yes	No	Yes	No
Yes	Yes	No	Yes	Yes	Yes	No	Yes	No
Yes	Yes	No	Yes	Yes	Yes	No	Yes	No
No	Yes	No	No	No	No	No	No	No
No	Yes	No	No	No	No	No	No	No
Yes	Yes	Yes	Yes	Yes	Yes	Yes	Yes	Yes
No	Yes	No	No	No	No	No	No	No
Yes	Yes	No	No	No	No	No	No	No
Yes	Yes	Yes	Yes	Yes	Yes	Yes	Yes	Yes

Table 2.4.0
Smoke-free legislation in the 100 biggest cities in the world

* Where population was recorded for both the city and urban agglomeration, the city population was used for reporting the cities by population size. Where the city population was missing but the urban agglomeration population was recorded the latter was used (respective cities are marked with an asterisk).

\# Smoke-free legislation adopted after 31 December 2008.

Please refer to Technical Note I for definition of complete smoke-free legislation.

CITY	POPULATION
Federal District (Mexico City)	18 204 965 *
Shanghai	14 348 535
Mumbai	11 978 450
Beijing	11 509 595
Sao Paulo	11 016 703
Istanbul	10 822 846 *
Moscow	10 456 490
Seoul	10 020 123
Delhi	9 879 172
Chongqing	9 691 901
Karachi	9 339 023
Jakarta	8 820 603
Guangzhou	8 524 826
Tokyo	8 489 653
Lima	8 445 211
Wuhan	8 312 700
London	8 278 251 *
New York	8 274 527
Tianjin	7 499 181
Tehran	7 088 287
Bogotá	7 050 228 *
Shenzhen	7 008 831
Hong Kong Special Administrative Region	6 925 900
Bangkok	6 842 000 *
Cairo	6 758 581
Dongguan	6 445 777
Rio De Janeiro	6 136 652
Toronto	5 509 874 *
Dhaka	5 333 571 *
Shenyang	5 303 053
Lagos	5 195 247
Lahore	5 143 495
Santiago	4 960 815
Singapore	4 588 600
Kolkata	4 572 876
Saint Petersburg	4 569 616
Xi'an	4 481 508
Chennai	4 343 645
Aleppo	4 337 000
Sydney	4 336 374
Chengdu	4 333 541
Bangalore	4 301 326
Riyadh	4 087 152
Ankara	3 953 344 *
Los Angeles	3 834 340
Guadalajara	3 833 866 *
Melbourne	3 806 092
Montréal	3 695 790 *
Hyderabad	3 637 483
Nanjing	3 624 234
Yokohama	3 579 628

Source: (*162*).

SMOKE-FREE LEGISLATION AS AT 31 DECEMBER 2008	COUNTRY
Covered by complete city-wide smoke-free legislation	Mexico
Not completely smoke-free	China
Not completely smoke-free	India
Not completely smoke-free	China
Covered by complete state-wide smoke-free legislation #	Brazil
Covered by complete national smoke-free legislation	Turkey
Not completely smoke-free	Russian Federation
Not completely smoke-free	Republic of Korea
Not completely smoke-free	India
Not completely smoke-free	China
Not completely smoke-free	Pakistan
Not completely smoke-free	Indonesia
Not completely smoke-free	China
Not completely smoke-free	Japan
Not completely smoke-free	Peru
Not completely smoke-free	China
Covered by complete national smoke-free legislation	United Kingdom of Great Britain and Northern Ireland
Covered by complete state-wide smoke-free legislation	United States of America
Not completely smoke-free	China
Covered by complete national smoke-free legislation	Iran (Islamic Republic of)
Covered by complete national smoke-free legislation	Colombia
Not completely smoke-free	China
Covered by complete city-wide smoke-free legislation	China
Not completely smoke-free	Thailand
Not completely smoke-free	Egypt
Not completely smoke-free	China
Covered by complete state-wide smoke-free legislation #	Brazil
Covered by complete state-wide smoke-free legislation	Canada
Not completely smoke-free	Bangladesh
Not completely smoke-free	China
Not completely smoke-free	Nigeria
Not completely smoke-free	Pakistan
Not completely smoke-free	Chile
Not completely smoke-free	Singapore
Not completely smoke-free	India
Not completely smoke-free	Russian Federation
Not completely smoke-free	China
Not completely smoke-free	India
Not completely smoke-free	Syrian Arab Republic
Covered by complete state-wide smoke-free legislation	Australia
Not completely smoke-free	China
Not completely smoke-free	India
Not completely smoke-free	Saudi Arabia
Covered by complete national smoke-free legislation	Turkey
Covered by complete state-wide smoke-free legislation	United States of America
Not completely smoke-free	Mexico
Covered by complete state-wide smoke-free legislation	Australia
Covered by complete state-wide smoke-free legislation	Canada
Not completely smoke-free	India
Not completely smoke-free	China
Not completely smoke-free	Japan

Table 2.4.0
Smoke-free legislation in the 100 biggest cities in the world

* Where population was recorded for both the city and urban agglomeration, the city population was used for reporting the cities by population size. Where the city population was missing but the urban agglomeration population was recorded the latter was used (respective cities are marked with an asterisk).

\# Smoke-free legislation adopted after 31 December 2008.

☆ Separate, completely enclosed smoking rooms are allowed if they are separately ventilated to the outside and kept under negative air pressure in relation to the surrounding areas. Given the difficulty of meeting the very strict requirements delineated for such rooms, they appear to be a practical impossibility but no reliable empirical evidence is presently available to ascertain whether they have been constructed.

Please refer to Technical Note I for definition of complete smoke-free legislation.

CITY	POPULATION
Busan	3 554 003
Ahmedabad	3 520 085
Haerbin	3 481 504
Monterrey	3 473 088 *
Berlin	3 386 667
Dalian	3 245 191
Changchun	3 225 557
Madrid	3 128 600
Kunming	3 035 406
Ho Chi Minh	3 015 743
Jinan	2 999 934
Casablanca	2 995 000
Guiyang	2 985 105
Buenos Aires	2 965 403
Nairobi	2 948 109
Chicago	2 836 658
Zibo	2 817 479
Jiddah	2 801 481
Pyongyang	2 741 260
Qingdao	2 720 972
Salvador	2 714 018
Kiev	2 676 789
Addis Ababa	2 646 000
Osaka	2 628 811
Rome	2 626 640
Surabaya	2 611 506
Incheon	2 596 317
Zhengzhou	2 589 387
Izmir	2 583 670 *
Taiyuan	2 558 382
Kanpur	2 551 337
Pune	2 538 473
Daegu	2 484 022
Chaoyang	2 470 812
Hangzhou	2 451 319
Surat	2 433 835
Mashhad	2 427 316
Fortaleza	2 416 920
Belo Horizonte	2 399 920
Brasilia	2 383 784
Zhongshan	2 363 322
Jaipur	2 322 575
Bandung	2 288 570
Vancouver	2 285 893 *
Medellín	2 264 776 *
Manchester	2 244 931 *
Nagoya	2 215 062
Houston	2 208 180
Guayaquil	2 194 442

Source: (162).

SMOKE-FREE LEGISLATION AS AT 31 DECEMBER 2008	COUNTRY
Not completely smoke-free	Republic of Korea
Not completely smoke-free	India
Not completely smoke-free	China
Not completely smoke-free	Mexico
Not completely smoke-free	Germany
Not completely smoke-free	China
Not completely smoke-free	China
Not completely smoke-free	Spain
Not completely smoke-free	China
Not completely smoke-free	Viet Nam
Not completely smoke-free	China
Not completely smoke-free	Morocco
Not completely smoke-free	China
Not completely smoke-free	Argentina
Not completely smoke-free	Kenya
Covered by complete state-wide smoke-free legislation	United States of America
Not completely smoke-free	China
Not completely smoke-free	Saudi Arabia
Not completely smoke-free	Democratic People's Republic of Korea
Not completely smoke-free	China
Covered by complete city-wide smoke-free legislation #	Brazil
Not completely smoke-free	Ukraine
Not completely smoke-free	Ethiopia
Not completely smoke-free	Japan
☆	Italy
Not completely smoke-free	Indonesia
Not completely smoke-free	Republic of Korea
Not completely smoke-free	China
Covered by complete national smoke-free legislation	Turkey
Not completely smoke-free	China
Not completely smoke-free	India
Not completely smoke-free	India
Not completely smoke-free	Republic of Korea
Not completely smoke-free	China
Not completely smoke-free	China
Not completely smoke-free	India
Covered by complete national smoke-free legislation	Iran (Islamic Republic of)
Not completely smoke-free	Brazil
Not completely smoke-free	Brazil
Not completely smoke-free	Brazil
Not completely smoke-free	China
Not completely smoke-free	India
Not completely smoke-free	Indonesia
Covered by complete state-wide smoke-free legislation	Canada
Covered by complete national smoke-free legislation	Colombia
Covered by complete national smoke-free legislation	United Kingdom of Great Britain and Northern Ireland
Not completely smoke-free	Japan
Not completely smoke-free	United States of America
Not completely smoke-free	Ecuador

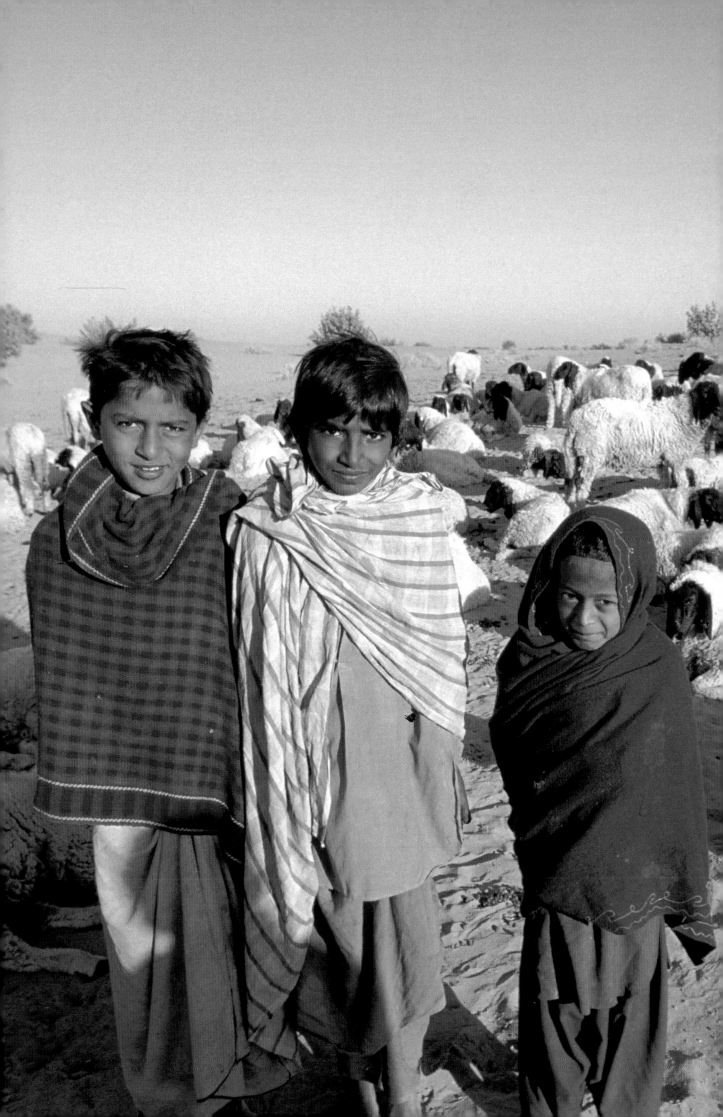

APPENDIX III: STATUS OF THE WHO FRAMEWORK CONVENTION ON TOBACCO CONTROL

Appendix III shows the status of the WHO Framework Convention on Tobacco Control (WHO FCTC). Ratification is the international act by which countries that have already signed a convention formally state their consent to be bound by it. Accession is the international act by which countries that have not signed a treaty/convention formally state their consent to be bound by it. Acceptance and approval are the legal equivalent of ratification. Signature of a convention indicates that a country is not legally bound by the treaty but is committed not to undermine its provisions.

The WHO FCTC entered into force on 27 February 2005, on the 90th day after the deposit of the 40th instrument of ratification in the United Nations headquarters, the depository of the treaty, in New York. The treaty remains open for ratification, acceptance, approval, formal confirmation and accession indefinitely for States and eligible regional economic integration organizations wishing to become Parties to it.

Table 3.1.0

Status of the WHO Framework Convention on Tobacco Control as of 22 October 2009

* Ratification is the international act by which countries that have already signed a treaty or convention formally state their consent to be bound by it.

ᵃ Accession is the international act by which countries that have not signed a treaty/convention formally state their consent to be bound by it.

ᴬ Acceptance is the international act, similar to ratification, by which countries that have already signed a treaty/convention formally state their consent to be bound by it.

ᴬᴬ Approval is the international act, similar to ratification, by which countries that have already signed a treaty/convention formally state their consent to be bound by it.

ᶜ Formal confirmation is the international act corresponding to ratification by a State, whereby an international organization (in the case of the WHO FCTC, competent regional economic integration organizations) formally state their consent to be bound by a treaty/convention.

ᵈ Succession is the international act, however phrased or named, by which successor States formally state their consent to be bound by treaties/conventions originally entered into by their predecessor State.

COUNTRY	DATE OF SIGNATURE	DATE OF RATIFICATION* (OR LEGAL EQUIVALENT)
Afghanistan	29 June 2004	
Albania	29 June 2004	26 April 2006
Algeria	20 June 2003	30 June 2006
Andorra		
Angola	29 June 2004	20 September 2007
Antigua and Barbuda	28 June 2004	5 June 2006
Argentina	25 September 2003	
Armenia		29 November 2004 ᵃ
Australia	5 December 2003	27 October 2004
Austria	28 August 2003	15 September 2005
Azerbaijan		1 November 2005 ᵃ
Bahamas	29 June 2004	
Bahrain		20 March 2007 ᵃ
Bangladesh	16 June 2003	14 June 2004
Barbados	28 June 2004	3 November 2005
Belarus	17 June 2004	8 September 2005
Belgium	22 January 2004	1 November 2005
Belize	26 September 2003	15 December 2005
Benin	18 June 2004	3 November 2005
Bhutan	9 December 2003	23 August 2004
Bolivia (Plurinational State of)	27 February 2004	15 September 2005
Bosnia and Herzegovina		10 July 2009
Botswana	16 June 2003	31 January 2005
Brazil	16 June 2003	3 November 2005
Brunei Darussalam	3 June 2004	3 June 2004
Bulgaria	22 December 2003	7 November 2005
Burkina Faso	22 December 2003	31 July 2006
Burundi	16 June 2003	22 November 2005
Cambodia	25 May 2004	15 November 2005
Cameroon	13 May 2004	3 February 2006
Canada	15 July 2003	26 November 2004
Cape Verde	17 February 2004	4 October 2005
Central African Republic	29 December 2003	7 November 2005
Chad	22 June 2004	30 January 2006
Chile	25 September 2003	13 June 2005
China	10 November 2003	11 October 2005
Colombia		10 April 2008 ᵃ
Comoros	27 February 2004	24 January 2006
Congo	23 March 2004	6 February 2007
Cook Islands	14 May 2004	14 May 2004
Costa Rica	3 July 2003	21 August 2008
Côte d'Ivoire	24 July 2003	
Croatia	2 June 2004	14 July 2008
Cuba	29 June 2004	
Cyprus	24 May 2004	26 October 2005
Czech Republic	16 June 2003	
Democratic People's Republic of Korea	17 June 2003	27 April 2005
Democratic Republic of the Congo	28 June 2004	28 October 2005
Denmark	16 June 2003	16 December 2004
Djibouti	13 May 2004	31 July 2005
Dominica	29 June 2004	24 July 2006

COUNTRY	DATE OF SIGNATURE	DATE OF RATIFICATION* (OR LEGAL EQUIVALENT)
Dominican Republic		
Ecuador	22 March 2004	25 July 2006
Egypt	17 June 2003	25 February 2005
El Salvador	18 March 2004	
Equatorial Guinea		17 September 2005 [a]
Eritrea		
Estonia	8 June 2004	27 July 2005
Ethiopia	25 February 2004	
European Community	16 June 2003	30 June 2005 [c]
Fiji	3 October 2003	3 October 2003
Finland	16 June 2003	24 January 2005
France	16 June 2003	19 October 2004 [AA]
Gabon	22 August 2003	20 February 2009
Gambia	16 June 2003	18 September 2007
Georgia	20 February 2004	14 February 2006
Germany	24 October 2003	16 December 2004
Ghana	20 June 2003	29 November 2004
Greece	16 June 2003	27 January 2006
Grenada	29 June 2004	14 August 2007
Guatemala	25 September 2003	16 November 2005
Guinea	1 April 2004	7 November 2007
Guinea-Bissau		7 November 2008 [a]
Guyana		15 September 2005 [a]
Haiti	23 July 2003	
Honduras	18 June 2004	16 February 2005
Hungary	16 June 2003	7 April 2004
Iceland	16 June 2003	14 June 2004
India	10 September 2003	5 February 2004
Indonesia		
Iran (Islamic Republic of)	16 June 2003	6 November 2005
Iraq	29 June 2004	17 March 2008
Ireland	16 September 2003	7 November 2005
Israel	20 June 2003	24 August 2005
Italy	16 June 2003	2 July 2008
Jamaica	24 September 2003	7 July 2005
Japan	9 March 2004	8 June 2004 A
Jordan	28 May 2004	19 August 2004
Kazakhstan	21 June 2004	22 January 2007
Kenya	25 June 2004	25 June 2004
Kiribati	27 April 2004	15 September 2005
Kuwait	16 June 2003	12 May 2006
Kyrgyzstan	18 February 2004	25 May 2006
Lao People's Democratic Republic	29 June 2004	6 September 2006
Latvia	10 May 2004	10 February 2005
Lebanon	4 March 2004	7 December 2005
Lesotho	23 June 2004	14 January 2005
Liberia	25 June 2004	15 September 2009
Libyan Arab Jamahiriya	18 June 2004	7 June 2005
Lithuania	22 September 2003	16 December 2004
Luxembourg	16 June 2003	30 June 2005
Madagascar	24 September 2003	22 September 2004

Table 3.1.0
Status of the WHO Framework Convention on Tobacco Control as of 22 October 2009

* Ratification is the international act by which countries that have already signed a treaty or convention formally state their consent to be bound by it.
a Accession is the international act by which countries that have not signed a treaty/convention formally state their consent to be bound by it.
A Acceptance is the international act, similar to ratification, by which countries that have already signed a treaty/convention formally state their consent to be bound by it.
AA Approval is the international act, similar to ratification, by which countries that have already signed a treaty/convention formally state their consent to be bound by it.
c Formal confirmation is the international act corresponding to ratification by a State, whereby an international organization (in the case of the WHO FCTC, competent regional economic integration organizations) formally state their consent to be bound by a treaty/convention
d Succession is the international act, however phrased or named, by which successor States formally state their consent to be bound by treaties/conventions originally entered into by their predecessor State

COUNTRY	DATE OF SIGNATURE	DATE OF RATIFICATION* (OR LEGAL EQUIVALENT)
Malawi		
Malaysia	23 September 2003	16 September 2005
Maldives	17 May 2004	20 May 2004
Mali	23 September 2003	19 October 2005
Malta	16 June 2003	24 September 2003
Marshall Islands	16 June 2003	8 December 2004
Mauritania	24 June 2004	28 October 2005
Mauritius	17 June 2003	17 May 2004
Mexico	12 August 2003	28 May 2004
Micronesia (Federated States of)	28 June 2004	18 March 2005
Monaco		
Mongolia	16 June 2003	27 January 2004
Montenegro		23 October 2006 [d]
Morocco	16 April 2004	
Mozambique	18 June 2003	
Myanmar	23 October 2003	21 April 2004
Namibia	29 January 2004	7 November 2005
Nauru		29 June 2004 [a]
Nepal	3 December 2003	7 November 2006
Netherlands	16 June 2003	27 January 2005 [A]
New Zealand	16 June 2003	27 January 2004
Nicaragua	7 June 2004	9 April 2008
Niger	28 June 2004	25 August 2005
Nigeria	28 June 2004	20 October 2005
Niue	18 June 2004	3 June 2005
Norway	16 June 2003	16 June 2003 [AA]
Oman		9 March 2005 [a]
Pakistan	18 May 2004	3 November 2004
Palau	16 June 2003	12 February 2004
Panama	26 September 2003	16 August 2004
Papua New Guinea	22 June 2004	25 May 2006
Paraguay	16 June 2003	26 September 2006
Peru	21 April 2004	30 November 2004
Philippines	23 September 2003	6 June 2005
Poland	14 June 2004	15 September 2006
Portugal	9 January 2004	8 November 2005 [AA]
Qatar	17 June 2003	23 July 2004
Republic of Korea	21 July 2003	16 May 2005
Republic of Moldova	29 June 2004	3 February 2009 [a]
Romania	25 June 2004	27 January 2006
Russian Federation		3 June 2008 [a]
Rwanda	2 June 2004	19 October 2005
Saint Kitts and Nevis	29 June 2004	
Saint Lucia	29 June 2004	7 November 2005
Saint Vincent and the Grenadines	14 June 2004	
Samoa	25 September 2003	3 November 2005
San Marino	26 September 2003	7 July 2004
Sao Tome and Principe	18 June 2004	12 April 2006
Saudi Arabia	24 June 2004	9 May 2005
Senegal	19 June 2003	27 January 2005
Serbia	28 June 2004	8 February 2006

COUNTRY	DATE OF SIGNATURE	DATE OF RATIFICATION* (OR LEGAL EQUIVALENT)
Seychelles	11 September 2003	12 November 2003
Sierra Leone		22 May 2009
Singapore	29 December 2003	14 May 2004
Slovakia	19 December 2003	4 May 2004
Slovenia	25 September 2003	15 March 2005
Solomon Islands	18 June 2004	10 August 2004
Somalia		
South Africa	16 June 2003	19 April 2005
Spain	16 June 2003	11 January 2005
Sri Lanka	23 September 2003	11 November 2003
Sudan	10 June 2004	31 October 2005
Suriname	24 June 2004	16 December 2008
Swaziland	29 June 2004	13 January 2006
Sweden	16 June 2003	7 July 2005
Switzerland	25 June 2004	
Syrian Arab Republic	11 July 2003	22 November 2004
Tajikistan		
Thailand	20 June 2003	8 November 2004
The former Yugoslav Republic of Macedonia		30 June 2006 [a]
Timor-Leste	25 May 2004	22 December 2004
Togo	12 May 2004	15 November 2005
Tonga	25 September 2003	8 April 2005
Trinidad and Tobago	27 August 2003	19 August 2004
Tunisia	22 August 2003	
Turkey	28 April 2004	31 December 2004
Turkmenistan		
Tuvalu	10 June 2004	26 September 2005
Uganda	5 March 2004	20 June 2007
Ukraine	25 June 2004	6 June 2006
United Arab Emirates	24 June 2004	7 November 2005
United Kingdom of Great Britain and Northern Ireland	16 June 2003	16 December 2004
United Republic of Tanzania	27 January 2004	30 April 2007
United States of America	10 May 2004	
Uruguay	19 June 2003	9 September 2004
Uzbekistan		
Vanuatu	22 April 2004	16 September 2005
Venezuela (Bolivarian Republic of)	22 September 2003	27 June 2006
Viet Nam	3 September 2003	17 December 2004
Yemen	20 June 2003	22 February 2007
Zambia		23 May 2008 [a]
Zimbabwe		

Source: WHO Framework Convention on Tobacco Control web site (http://www.who.int/fctc/signatories_parties/, accessed 26 October 2009).

Though not a Member State of WHO, as a Member State of the United Nations, Liechtenstein is also eligible to become Party to the WHO FCTC, though it has taken no action to do so.

On submitting instruments to become Party to the WHO FCTC, some Parties have included notes and/or declarations. All notes can be viewed at http://www.who.int/fctc/signatories_parties/. All declarations can be viewed at http://www.who.int/fctc/declarations/en/index.html.

Acknowledgments

The following WHO staff assisted in compiling, analysing and editing information:

WHO African Region:
Jean-Pierre Baptiste, Tecla Butau, Deowan Mohee, Nivo Ramanandraibe.

WHO Region of the Americas:
Adriana Blanco, Maristela Monteiro, Rosa Sandoval, Mayte Vasquez.

WHO South-East Asia Region:
Khalil Rahman, Kamar Rezwan, Dhirendra N. Sinha.

WHO European Region:
Yulia Kadirova, Rula Khoury, Kristina Mauer, Agis Tsouros.

WHO Eastern Mediterranean Region:
Fatimah El-Awa, Majed Elehawi, Farrukh Qureshi.

WHO Western Pacific Region:
Sarah England (China), Trinette Lee, Guangyuan Liu, Susan Mercado.

WHO-Headquarters Geneva:
Sundus Aladoofi, Zahra Ali Piazza, Ala Alwan, Alphaluck Bhatiasevi, Lubna Bhatti, Douglas Bettcher, Katherine DeLand, Christine Fares, Daniel Ferrante, Gillian Forbes, Omid Fotuhi, Dongbo Fu, Lejla Gagic, Bernardus Ganter, Jason Henderson, Gudrun Ingolfsdottir, Mie Inoue, Sun Goo Lee, Nima Mansouri, Raman Minhas, Ryan Moran, Simeon Niles, Timothy O'Leary, Alexandre Pascutto, Armando Peruga, Patrick Petit (formerly WHO), Luminita Sanda, Rosane Serrao, Brooke Trainum, Gulnoza Usmanova, Barbara Zolty.

Administrative support was provided by: Miriamjoy Aryee-Quansah, Catalin Iacobescu, Luis Madge, Carolyn Patten, Elizabeth Tecson, Jennifer Volonnino.

Kerstin Schotte coordinated the production of this report with support from Katherine DeLand.

Christopher Fitzpatrick provided technical oversight to the development of its content.

Quality assurance of country-reported data was assured by Alison Commar, Christopher Fitzpatrick, Gauri Khanna, Sameer Pujari, Kerstin Schotte and Erin Smith.

Armando Peruga was responsible for the legal review process performed by: Dongbo Fu, Raman Minhas, Luminita Sanda, Erin Smith, Gemma Vestal and Barbara Zolty.

The prevalence estimates were calculated by Gauri Khanna and Edouard Tursan d'Espaignet.

The financial and economic review and analyses, including tobacco taxation and prices, were provided by Christopher Fitzpatrick (AFR and SEAR), Anne-Marie Perucic (AMR and EMR) and Ayda Yurekli (EUR and WPR) with support from Frank Chaloupka and Sofia Delipalla.

Data management, quality assurance and creation of tables, graphs and appendices were performed by Alison Commar, Sameer Pujari and Shaun Takao.

We thank Jennifer Ellis and Kelly Henning of the Bloomberg Initiative to Reduce Tobacco Use for their collaboration. Stella Bialous, Vera da Costa e Silva, Geoffrey T. Fong, John Pierce, Martin Raw and Jonathan Samet, among others, provided us with invaluable feedback and comments, thank you very much. Special thanks also to the Convention Secretariat to the WHO FCTC, to Colin Mathers and Gretchen Stevens, and to the team of the Office on Smoking and Health of the US Centers for Disease Control and Prevention (CDC).

Drew Blakeman assisted with the drafting of this report. Special thanks are due to our copyeditor and proofreader Barbara Campanini and our designer Reda Sadki and his team for their efficiency in helping to get this report published in time.

Production of this WHO document has been supported by a grant from the World Lung Foundation with financial support from Bloomberg Philanthropies. The contents of this document are the sole responsibility of WHO and should not be regarded as reflecting the positions of the World Lung Foundation.

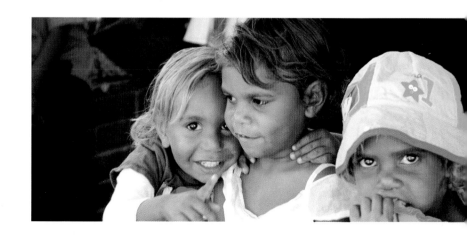